Assessment of Risk in the Term Newborn, 2nd Edition

Carole Kenner, DNS, RNC-NIC, FAAN
Leslie Altimier, MSN, RNC

Editor
Rita Reis Wieczorek, EdD, RN, PNP, FAAN

Consulting Editor
Margaret Comerford Freda, EdD, RN, CHES, FAAN

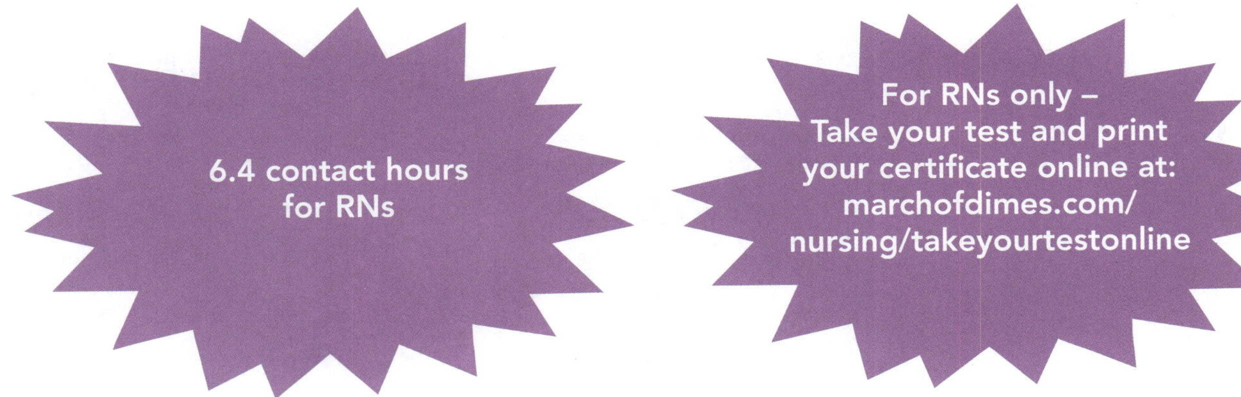

33-2294-08 8/08
ISBN 0-86525-122-9

Library of Congress Cataloging-in-Publication Data

Kenner, Carole.
  Assessment of risk in the term newborn. -- 2nd ed. / Carole Kenner, Leslie Altimier ; editor, Rita Reis Wieczorek ; consulting editor, Margaret Comerford Freda.
       p. ; cm.
  Rev. ed. of: Assessment of risk in the term newborn / Susan Bakewell-Sachs, Valerie D. Shaw, Amy L. Tashman. c1997.
  Includes bibliographical references.
  ISBN 978-0-86525-122-9
  1. Newborn infants–Health risk assessment–Programmed instruction. 2. Pediatric nursing–Programmed instruction. 3. Newborn infants–Diseases–Diagnosis–Programmed instruction. I. Altimier, Leslie. II. Wieczorek, Rita Reis. III. Bakewell-Sachs, Susan. Assessment of risk in the term newborn. IV. March of Dimes Birth Defects Foundation. Education & Health Promotion Dept. V. Title.
  [DNLM: 1. Neonatal Nursing–Programmed Instruction. 2. Infant, Newborn. 3. Nursing Assessment–Programmed Instruction. 4. Risk Factors–Programmed Instruction. WY 18.2 K36a 2008]
  RJ255.6.H4B35 2008
  618.92'01--dc22

2008019476

Published by:
Education & Health Promotion
March of Dimes

Editor
Rita Reis Wieczorek, EdD, RN, PNP, FAAN
Manager, Nursing Outreach and Education
March of Dimes

Associate Editor
Karen Kroder
Director, Educational Print Materials
March of Dimes

Assistant Editor
Jackie Frankel
Assistant Manager, Professional Education
Materials and Services
March of Dimes

Project Manager
Mary Lavan
Manager, Professional Education Services
March of Dimes

The March of Dimes is a national voluntary health agency whose mission is to improve the health of babies by preventing birth defects, premature birth and infant mortality. Founded in 1938, the March of Dimes funds programs of research, community services, education and advocacy to save babies and, in 2003, launched a campaign to address the increasing rate of premature birth. For more information, visit the March of Dimes Web site at marchofdimes.com or in Spanish at nacersano.org.

Part of the March of Dimes educational objective includes producing high-quality, low-cost educational resources for health care providers including March of Dimes nursing modules; assessment tools designed to enhance the skills of professionals who work with pregnant women; and videos and brochures to help providers communicate key reproductive health messages to clients.

Some March of Dimes publications may, on occasion, contain controversial views. All such statements and opinions are the sole responsibility of the authors and do not reflect an endorsement by the March of Dimes or the editors unless expressly stated.

March of Dimes materials reflect current scientific recommendations at time of publication. These recommendations may change. Please check marchofdimes.com for updated information.

To order additional copies of this or any March of Dimes nursing module or to request a free March of Dimes continuing education catalog, contact:

March of Dimes Fulfillment Center
P.O. Box 932852
Atlanta, GA 31193-2852
Phone: 800-367-6630
Fax: 770-280-4116

For further information on March of Dimes nursing modules, contact:

March of Dimes
Education & Health Promotion
1275 Mamaroneck Avenue
White Plains, NY 10605
Phone: 914-997-4609
E-mail: profedu@marchofdimes.com
Web site: marchofdimes.com/nursing

Assessment of Risk in the Term Newborn, 2nd Edition

Tables and Figures

Module Topics

Nursing modules are self-directed learning monographs written by expert nurses for nursing professionals who provide care for women and infants. Each module addresses a specific topic and provides practical clinical information. Topics range from preconception to the neonatal period and cover changes that occur during the transition from intrauterine to extrauterine life; care of the pregnant woman an her fetus; the labor and delivery period; care of the postpartum woman and her neonate; and current and future critical perinatal health problems. Modules provide background information and caregiving standards to meet these issues and address assessment of risk, stabilization of the client and emergency care.

Nursing modules do not supplant didactic educational and clinical experiences. Rather, they are designed to provide registered nurses with information to enhance their baseline skills. Learners may require various levels of guidance to apply the materials to practice; for modules that deal with advanced practice topics, clinical application may initially require close supervision.

The March of Dimes recognizes the need to incorporate new, practical information and theoretical knowledge into nursing practice. To meet this challenge and promote excellent care for mothers and infants, the March of Dimes regularly convenes its Nurse Advisory Council to evaluate the nursing modules, to determine their direction and to recommend development of new titles addressing vital issues confronting nurses today.

How to Use March of Dimes Nursing Modules

1. Read the *Cognitive Objectives, Expected Practice Outcomes* and *Key Concepts*.

2. Take the *Pre-/Postinstructional Measurement* to assess your knowledge of the subject.

3. Read the module.

4. Complete the *Clinical Application*. In a group setting, the facilitator arranges a meeting to discuss the *Clinical Application* and *Group Discussion Items*.

5. Review the *References, Guidelines Related to This Topic* and *Supplementary Materials* to reinforce the module content and its use in clinical practice.

6. Repeat the *Pre-/Postinstructional Measurement* to assess learning.

7. To obtain CNE credit, follow the instructions for independent study or facilitated group study.

Continuing Nursing Education (CNE)

March of Dimes Accreditation

The March of Dimes is an approved provider of continuing nursing education by the New York State Nurses Association, an accredited approver of continuing nursing education by the American Nurses Credentialing Center's (ANCC) Commission on Accreditation.

It has been assigned code 6R2GNS-PRV-06.

The March of Dimes also is approved by the California Board of Registered Nursing, Provider #CEP11444.

This module is valid for **6.4 contact hours**. Note that in compliance with ANCC's criteria for CNE providers, contact hours provided by the March of Dimes are based on a 60-minute contact hour. Before January 1, 2007, the March of Dimes based contact hours on a 50-minute contact hour; therefore, all nursing module contact hours have been recalculated and certificates of completion reflect the change. Contact the Manager of Professional Education Services at 914.997.4609 with any questions.

The March of Dimes has submitted this module to the American College of Nurse-Midwives (ACNM) for approval of continuing education units (CEUs) for certified nurse-midwives (CNMs). CNMs should check the March of Dimes Web site at marchofdimes.com/ nursing to verify approval status. ACNM approval expires 2 years after the module's approval date. CNMs should verify the module's approval status with the March of Dimes if used after the 2-year expiration.

For the most up-to-date information about earning CNE credit and nursing modules, go to marchofdimes.com/nursing.

To qualify for CNE credit, participants must successfully complete a nursing module via independent study or facilitated group study.

Independent Study

Participants can earn CNE credit in the following ways:

1. Complete and submit the **original** *Independent Study Application* from the module and the *Module Evaluation*. No additional fee is required.

2. Take the test and complete the *Module Evaluation* online at marchofdimes.com/nursing/takeyourtestonline. Online tests require a **$15 fee payable by credit card.**

3. Complete and submit a **photocopy** of the module's *Independent Study Application* and the *Module Evaluation* with a **$15 check** made payable to the March of Dimes.

4. **Download** the module's *Independent Study Application* and the *Module Evaluation* from marchofdimes.com/nursing. Complete and submit the application and evaluation with a **$15 check** made payable to the March of Dimes.

Participants should mail *Independent Study Applications* and fees, when applicable to:

March of Dimes Nursing Modules
1275 Mamaroneck Avenue
White Plains, NY 10605

The March of Dimes notifies participants of test results within 4 weeks of receiving the completed application. Participants with scores of 70 percent or higher receive a certificate of completion; participants with scores <70 percent are offered a second attempt to pass the test.

The module purchase price includes one set of contact hours. There is no additional fee when using the **original** *Independent Study Application*. Participants choosing to share a module can obtain contact hours by taking the test online or mailing a completed **copy** of the *Independent Study Application* to the March of Dimes with a check for $15.

Independent Study Test

To receive CNE credit for this module via independent study, record your answers to the following questions on the *Independent Study Application* and follow the submission instructions.

For RNs only: Take your test online at marchofdimes.com/nursing/takeyourtestonline. This is the fastest way to take the test and receive a certificate.

1. A newborn's assessment reveals a heart rate of 104, a weak cry, some flexion of the extremities, a grimace when stimulated and pale body color. The newborn's Apgar score is:
    A. 4
    B. 5
    C. 6
    D. 7

2. Evidenced-based practice refers to the use of:
    A. Research findings
    B. Written guidelines
    C. Traditional practices
    D. Institutional policies

3. A newborn weighs 1,750 g at 36 weeks of gestation. This newborn is identified as:
    A. Term appropriate
    B. Preterm
    C. Small for gestational age (SGA)
    D. Appropriate for gestational age (AGA)

4. A newborn weighs 1,250 g at 34 weeks of gestation. A complication the nurse should watch for is:
    A. Decreased red blood cells
    B. Cephalohematoma
    C. Hypoglycemia
    D. Birth injuries

5. In an assessment for neuromuscular maturity in a newborn, a full-term neonate may be expected to:
    A. Fully extend extremities while lying
    B. Flex the wrist completely against the forearm
    C. Move the foot toward the head with a fully extended knee
    D. Move the arm toward the opposite shoulder with the elbow past the midline

6. Metabolic screening of newborns is primarily performed because:
    A. There is an increased incidence of metabolic problems in newborns.
    B. Diagnostic procedures are easier to perform in the hospital.
    C. Screening programs are mandatory in most states.
    D. Early treatment can prevent disability.

7. To prevent heat loss in the newborn via conduction, the nurse should:
    A. Maintain room temperature at 24 C.
    B. Swaddle the newborn with a blanket.
    C. Place the newborn on a warm surface.
    D. Dry the newborn immediately after bathing.

8. The nurse places a newborn's bassinette near the wall opposite a window. By this intervention, the nurse is preventing heat loss through:
    A. Evaporation
    B. Convection
    C. Conduction
    D. Radiation

9. While caring for a newborn who is at risk of developing hyperglycemia, the nurse should monitor the newborn for signs of:
    A. Cardiac dysrhythmias
    B. Respiratory distress
    C. Ineffective feeding
    D. Osmotic diuresis

10. A 2-day-old newborn's hematocrit is 70 percent and is diagnosed with polycythemia. The initial intervention that the practitioner may order to lower the hematocrit is:
    A. Phototherapy
    B. Increased fluid intake
    C. Insulin administration
    D. Partial exchange transfusion

11. The nurse identifies that an 8-hour-old is not jaundiced and has no associated risk factors for hyperbilirubinemia. The nurse should:
    A. Place the newborn unclothed near a sunny window.
    B. Encourage breastfeeding every 1½ hours for 48 hours.
    C. Obtain a blood sample for a total serum bilirubin level every 12 hours.
    D. Assess the newborn for jaundice every 8 hours until discharge.

12. Which adaptation by a neonate supports the presence of syphilis?
    A. Large for gestational age (LGA)
    B. Ruddy, purplish color
    C. Increased number of red blood cells
    D. Vesicular eruptions on the soles of the feet

13. A woman at 40 weeks gestation is in labor. She expels amniotic fluid that has evidence of meconium. After birth, the neonate has bradycardia, depressed respirations and flaccidity. What is the nurse's first intervention?
    A. Dry the neonate thoroughly.
    B. Perform endotracheal suctioning.
    C. Stimulate the soles of the neonate's feet.
    D. Aspirate mucous from the neonate's nose with a bulb syringe.

14. The nurse is teaching a group of parents about approaches to prevent sudden infant death syndrome (SIDS). The nurse identifies that additional teaching is necessary when a mother states, "I should:
    A. "Use a light blanket over, rather than under, my baby."
    B. "Put my baby to sleep on a firm, rather than a soft, sleep surface."
    C. "Sleep in the same room as my baby, rather than a separate room."
    D. "Place my baby on his back, rather than his stomach, when sleeping."

15. The nurse performs an abdominal assessment on a newborn. Which assessment may indicate a major health problem?
    A. Absence of a palpable spleen
    B. Pearly white, gelatinous umbilical cord
    C. Umbilical cord with two arteries and one vein
    D. Liver located 3.5 cm below the right costal margin

16. The nurse assesses the head of a newborn born via a vertex presentation. Which newborn assessment should the nurse immediately report to the practitioner?
    A. A posterior fontanel that is one cm wide
    B. The presence of caput succedaneum
    C. An anterior fontanel that is tense
    D. Overlapping skull sutures

17. The nurse observes a newborn in the transitional nursery. The nurse expects the newborn to enter the period of relative inactivity:
    A. One hour after birth
    B. Two to 3 hours after birth
    C. Four to 5 hours after birth
    D. Six hours after birth

18. Before administering the ordered dose of vitamin K to a newborn, the nurse must consider that:
    A. It must be administered intramuscularly.
    B. It should be given in the deltoid muscle.
    C. It should be given after circumcision.
    D. It must be administered after the result of a partial thromboplastin time is reviewed.

19. A newborn receives phototherapy with fluorescent lamps for moderate jaundice. It is most important that the nurse:
    A. Position the newborn at a distance of 24 inches from the lamps.
    B. Monitor newborns with extreme serum bilirubin levels every 1 to 2 hours.
    C. Monitor the newborn for signs of dehydration.
    D. Assess the newborn for signs of constipation.

20. The nurse understands that developmental care is based on the premise that:
    A. Infants require individualized care.
    B. Infants require common care approaches as they develop.
    C. Nurses initially are the primary providers of care for infants.
    D. Nurses should provide care based on the infant's gestational age.

Facilitated Group Study (Workshop/Grand Rounds/Conference)

A facilitated group study requires facilitation by a qualified registered nurse. A facilitated group study may occur as an in-service education program, as a workshop or nursing grand rounds, or as a portion of a larger conference or educational meeting. To earn CNE credit for this module via facilitated group study, each participant must:

1. Complete the module.

2. Participate in the facilitated group study.

3. Provide first and last name and mailing address.

4. Complete the *Module Evaluation* and submit it to the facilitator.

The facilitator must:

1. Be an RN.

2. Arrange time and location for the group study.

3. Facilitate discussion on the content of the module, as well as the *Clinical Application* and *Group Discussion Items*.

4. Register as a group study facilitator by sending an e-mail to certificate@ marchofdimes.com with facilitator name, organization name, mailing address and telephone number.

5. After receiving a confirmation e-mail reply, register the group study and participants and print certificates online at the March of Dimes Nursing Module Certificate Center. The e-mail confirmation provides the Center's Web address and password. Required registration information includes module title; study date, location and facilitator; and participant names and addresses. Use the participant roster on the next page to record participant names and addresses.

6. Collect *Module Evaluation* from participants and return to March of Dimes.

7. Distribute certificates of completion to participants.

For additional information, contact:

March of Dimes Education & Health Promotion
Telephone: 914-997-4609
Fax: 914-997-4501
E-mail: profedu@marchofdimes.com
Web site: marchofdimes.com/nursing

Facilitated Group Study Participant Roster

Assessment of Risk in the Term Newborn, 2nd Edition

Facilitator ___________________________________   **Date** _______________________

Location ____

Use this sign-in sheet to record participation in the facilitated group study.

	First Name	Last Name	Mailing Address	City	State	ZIP
1						
2						
3						
4						
5						
6						
7						
8						
9						
10						
11						
12						
13						
14						
15						
16						
17						
18						
19						
20						

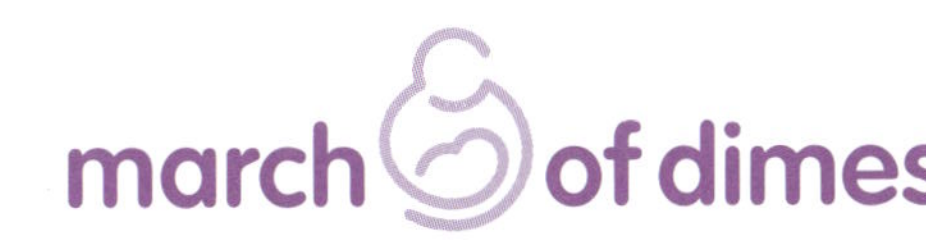

Editor's Acknowledgements

Special thanks to authors **Carole Kenner, DNS, RNC-NIC, FAAN** and
Leslie Altimier, MSN, RNC for making their knowledge available to nurses and
health care providers through the publication of this module.

Additional thanks to our consulting editor:

Margaret Comerford Freda, EdD, RN, CHES, FAAN
Professor, Department of Obstetrics, Gynecology and Women's Health
Albert Einstein College of Medicine
Montefiore Medical Center
Bronx, New York

We also gratefully acknowledge the following reviewer who so generously shared
her expertise.

Susan Rumsey Givens, MPH, RNC, LCCE
Childbirth Educator
Mt. Carmel St. Ann's Hospital
Westerville, Ohio

About This Module

Assessment of Risk in the Term Newborn, 2nd Edition provides perinatal and
neonatal health care providers with essential, evidence-based information to assess
a newborn's physiologic adaptation to extrauterine life and to assess for infectious
or metabolic disorders and positively support development. Gestational age
assessment, physical assessment and newborn behavior patterns are discussed. The
module outlines nursing management during the early newborn period, including
identification of risk factors and assessment, monitoring and intervention during
hospitalization and postdischarge follow-up.

Authors

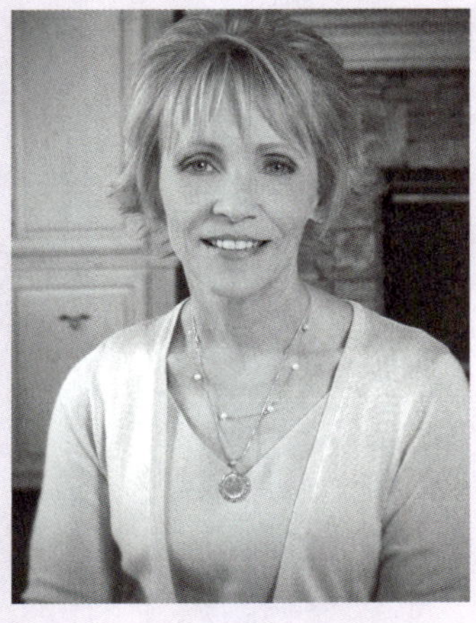

Carole Kenner

BSN, University of Cincinnati, Cincinnati, Ohio
MSN, Indiana University, Indianapolis, Indiana
DNS, Indiana University, Indianapolis, Indiana

Carole Kenner is dean and professor at the University of Oklahoma Health Sciences Center College of Nursing, Oklahoma City, Oklahoma. Her clinical background includes neonatal intensive care, genetics, palliative care and home follow-up care of high-risk infants and their families. Her primary research interest focuses on transition from hospital to home for mothers and babies, perinatal substance abuse, genetics and palliative/end-of-life care.

Dr. Kenner is president of the Council of International Neonatal Nurses (COINN), past president of the National Association of Neonatal Nurses (NAAN), past secretary and a fellow of the American Academy of Nursing (AAN), and a member of the March of Dimes Nurse Advisory Council, the Association of Women's Health, Obstetric and Neonatal Nurses (AWHONN), the Society of Pediatric Nurses, Sigma Theta Tau International and the National Organization of Nurse Practitioner Faculties (NONPF). She is certified in neonatal care through NCC.

Dr. Kenner has (a) no relationship with companies who manufacture products used in the treatment of the subjects under discussion; (b) no relationship with commercial supporter(s) of this activity and (c) no intent to discuss unlabeled uses of a commercial product, or an investigational use of a product not yet approved for this purpose.

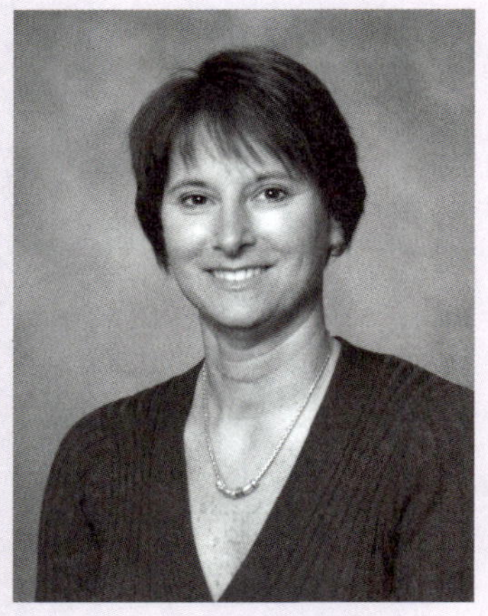

Leslie Altimier

BSN, Kent State University, Kent, Ohio
MSN, University of North Carolina, Greensboro, North Carolina

Ms. Altimier is the director of Women & Children Services at Mercy Hospital Anderson in Cincinnati, Ohio. In her nursing career of 20+ years, she has worked in neurosurgical, pediatric and neonatal intensive care units, a family birth center and in women's health. Her primary interest focuses on developmentally appropriate family-centered care. She has contributed to nursing through practice, education, leadership and research. She is certified in nursing administration through ANCC.

Ms. Altimier is author of NANN (National Association of Neonatal Nurses) *Guidelines for Neonatal Nursing Policies, Procedures, Competencies, and Clinical Pathways*, 4th Edition (Altimier, Brown & Tedeschi, 2006) and *Mosby's Neonatal Nursing Online Course* (2007), an innovative neonatal orientation program. She is the editor of *Newborn and Infant Nursing Reviews* (NAINR); president of Preemie Creations (www.preemiecreations.com), an online clearinghouse of information for parents of premature babies; and a member of AWHONN, the International Academy of Nurse Editors (INANE) and NANN. She also chairs NANN's Education Provider Committee and is on the Developmental Credential Task Force.

Ms. Altimier has (a) no relationship with companies who manufacture products used in the treatment of the subjects under discussion; (b) no relationship with commercial supporter(s) of this activity and (c) no intent to discuss unlabeled uses of a commercial product, or an investigational use of a product not yet approved for this purpose.

Cognitive Objectives

Upon completion of this module, the learner will be able to:

1. Describe evidence-based practice and developmental care as they related to neonatal care, growth and development.

2. Describe the five components of the Apgar score.

3. Describe the process of conducting a gestational assessment and the implications for care.

4. Discuss the differences between small for gestational age (SGA), appropriate for gestational age (AGA) and large for gestational age (LGA) and their implications for care.

5. Describe the use of the family history tool and how it fits with genetic testing and newborn screening.

6. Describe how to conduct a physical assessment, including gestational assessment and growth classifications.

7. Discuss newborn behavioral states during transition to extrauterine life.

8. Describe the four methods of newborn heat loss.

9. Identify nursing management strategies to prevent cold stress.

10. Identify risk factors, symptoms and management of common neonatal respiratory, hematologic and metabolic problems and problems transitioning to extrauterine life.

11. Describe newborns at risk for polycythemia management.

12. Identify the most common pathogens that cause perinatal and neonatal infections.

13. Discuss the significance of glycemic control and the risk factors for hyper- or hypoglycemia.

14. Describe follow-up care, including assessment for safety and abuse.

Expected Practice Outcomes

The learner who meets the objectives and understands the key concepts of this module can be expected to:

1. Apply evidence-based practice guidelines to newborn and family care.

2. Assign an appropriate Apgar score to a newborn.

3. Determine gestational age and classify as small for gestational age (SGA), appropriate for gestational age (AGA) or large for gestational age (LGA), based on physical and neurological assessments.

4. Conduct a newborn physical assessment.

5. Assess infant state.

6. Obtain specimens for genetic and metabolic newborn screening.

7. Apply thermoregulation concepts in caring for the neonate.

8. Describe the nurse's role in the care of an infant with common respiratory, hematologic, metabolic problems or with problems transitioning to extrauterine life.

9. Eliminate factors that predispose the newborn to hypoglycemia.

10. Monitor the newborn for signs and symptoms of infection.

11. Assess the newborn for risk of polycythemia.

12. Manage symptoms associated with physiologic and nonphysiologic jaundice.

13. Manage the infant on phototherapy.

14. Assess for risk factors for abuse.

Key Concepts

The material in this module will help the learner understand the following concepts:

1. Newborns follow a predictable set of behaviors as they transition to extrauterine life.

2. The Apgar score indicates the need for resuscitation, but not the degree of asphyxia or the neurologic potential.

3. The gestational age exam is a tool to determine risk factors and plan appropriate nursing care.

4. Newborn heat loss can occur through four mechanisms: conduction, convection, radiation and evaporation.

5. Gestational age is the most predictive criterion for survival of the newborn.

6. Inappropriate management of cold stress and heat stress in neonates is associated with metabolic complications, such as hypoglycemia, increased oxygen consumption, increased lactic acid production, increased metabolic acidosis and death.

7. Symptoms of hypoglycemia may be absent despite extremely low blood glucose levels.

8. Prevention is the best method of treatment for neonatal viral and bacterial infection.

9. Treatment of polycythemia is controversial and is usually not provided unless symptoms are present.

10. Infants with extreme hyperbilirubinemia are at risk for developing bilirubin encephalopathy and acute bilirubin encephalopathy (ABE).

11. Therapeutic management of the newborn with hyperbilirubinemia is based on clinical judgment, history, course and clinical findings.

12. Nurses can identify risk factors for and symptoms of newborn abuse at discharge or in initial follow-up visits.

Guidelines Related to This Topic

The following guidelines provide additional information and instructions on the module topic.

Author, Year	Guideline	Source
American Academy of Pediatrics (AAP), 2002	Perinatal asphyxia	www.aap.org
AAP, 2004	Management of hyperbilirubinemia in the newborn infant 35 or more weeks of gestation	aappolicy.aappublications.org/cgi/content/full/pediatrics;114/1/297
AAP, 2006	Neonatal resuscitation	www.app.org/nrp/nrpmain.html
American College of Medical Genetics, 2006	Newborn screening ACT sheets and confirmatory algorithms	www.acmg.net/resources/policies/ACT/condition-analyte-links.htm
American Nurses Association (ANA) & NANN, 2004	Neonatal nursing scope and standards of practice	www.nursingworld.org www.nann.org
Association for Women's Health, Obstetric and Neonatal Nursing (AWHONN), 2006	Emerging issues in near-term infant care	www.awhonn.org
AWHONN & NANN, 1998	Neonatal skin care	www.awhonn.org/awhonn/store/productDetail.do?productCode=ENSC-2
Centers for Disease Control and Prevention (CDC), 2006	Group B strep prevention	www.cdc.gov/groupBstrep/news/news_guidelines_summary.htm
CDC, 2006	Sexually transmitted diseases	www.cdc.gov/mmwr/preview/mmwrhtml/rr5511a1.htm
Sixth Consensus Conference on Newborn ICU Design, 2006	Newborn intensive care unit design	www.nd.edu/~nicudes/Recommended%20Standards%205.10%20pdf.pdf

Pre-/Postinstructional Measurement

Choose the best response to each question. Check your answer with the key.

1. A newborn's assessment reveals a heart rate of 140, loud crying, some flexion of the arms and legs, withdrawal of the feet when stimulated and a pink body with blue extremities. The newborn's Apgar score is:
   A. 5
   B. 6
   C. 7
   D. 8

2. A newborn weighs 3,790 g at 40 weeks of gestation. This newborn is identified as:
   A. Appropriate for gestational age (AGA)
   B. Large for gestational age (LGA)
   C. Post-term
   D. Preterm

3. A complication of LGA that the nurse should watch for is:
   A. Facial nerve palsy
   B. Congenital heart defect
   D. Elevated blood glucose
   C. Increased red blood cells

4. The nurse understands that the ideal time to obtain samples for newborn screening tests is:
   A. Four days after birth
   B. Six hours after birth
   C. Between 48 hours and 72 hours after birth
   D. Between 12 hours and 24 hours after birth

5. A laboring woman gives birth to a healthy, full-term neonate in the birthing suite. The nurse dries the newborn to reduce body heat loss through the mechanism of:
   A. Radiation
   B. Convection
   C. Conduction
   D. Evaporation

6. To prevent heat loss in the newborn via radiation, the nurse should:
   A. Bathe the newborn in warm water.
   B. Place a head covering on the newborn.
   C. Dry the newborn immediately after a bath.
   D. Put a cloth covering on the scale before weighing a newborn.

7. The nurse assesses a newborn for signs of cold stress. Which adaptation is unrelated to cold stress?
   A. Decreased serum glucose
   B. Increased metabolic acidosis
   C. Increased oxygen consumption
   D. Decreased lactic acid production

8. The primary heat production mechanism in the newborn is:
   A. Decreasing oxygen consumption
   B. Metabolizing brown fat
   C. Shivering
   D. Sweating

9. The most common metabolic complication found in polycythemia is:
   A. Polyuria
   B. Bradycardia
   C. Hypoglycemia
   D. Hypercalcemia

10. The nurse monitors a newborn for signs of jaundice. What area of the body should the nurse expect signs of jaundice to be exhibited first?
    A. Back
    B. Chest
    C. Forehead
    D. Extremities

11. The nurse performs a physical assessment of the newborn. Which sign supports the presence of ophthalmia neonatorum?
    A. Rhinitis
    B. Jaundice
    C. Hyperthermia
    D. Conjunctivitis

12. During the initial period of reactivity, which assessment may require immediate intervention?
    A. Presence of acrocyanosis
    B. Heart rate of 160 beats per minute
    C. Asymmetrical chest wall movements
    D. Respirations of 50 breaths per minute

13. A newborn has an electrode secured with an adhesive. The nurse should remove the adhesive by:
    A. Using cotton soaked in mineral oil
    B. Rubbing with an alcohol swab
    C. Waiting 12 hours after it is applied
    D. Soaking it with a solvent

14. The nurse is teaching a parenting class about child abuse. The factor most related to the potential for child abuse is that:
    A. The family has members of 3 generations living in one house.
    B. The mother is the primary caretaker of the infant.
    C. The parents have a high socioeconomic status.
    D. The father is inexperienced with child care.

15. The nurse performs an initial skin assessment of a newborn. Which observation is most important to report:
    A. Multiple, large, brown-pigmented spots on the body
    B. Blue, bruise-like macular spots on the sacrum
    C. Pinhead-sized, whitish papules on the face
    D. Waxy, whitish substance on skin folds

ASSESSMENT OF RISK IN THE TERM NEWBORN, 2nd Edition

Carole Kenner, DNS, RNC-NIC, FAAN
Leslie Altimier, MSN, RNC

Transition from Fetal to Extrauterine Life

Changes in organ-system functions and reorganization of metabolic processes require movement from fetal patterns of circulation to establishment of pulmonary gas exchange resembling an adult cardiovascular pattern and a stable serum glucose level. The newborn also must maintain body temperature and break down excess red blood cells (RBCs). While most term newborns achieve physiologic homeostasis without complications, assessment and monitoring of neonatal adaptation are essential for early identification of problems, including cold stress, hypoglycemia, infection, polycythemia and hyperbilirubinemia. Vitamin K administration, eye prophylaxis and routine screening for genetic and metabolic diseases help prevent and identify conditions that threaten the health and well-being of newborns. The perinatal history, including maternal, paternal, antepartal and intrapartal data, gives perinatal and neonatal nurses important baseline information regarding newborn risk (Barron, 2007). Gestational age and anthropometric and physical assessment data, along with newborn behavior, provide further evidence of risk and well-being. Nursing management during the early newborn period includes identification of risk factors, assessment, monitoring, intervention and postdischarge follow-up.

Evidence-based Practice and Developmental Care

Evidence-based practice (EBP) is based on the concept that care is grounded in research findings, rather than experience and tradition. EBP is a problem-solving approach in which health care providers critically appraise research findings and make decisions about using the findings in practice (Theroux, 2006). EBP enables nurses to provide the highest quality of care in meeting the multifaceted needs of newborns and their families. When nurses and other health care providers can find, critically appraise and use the best evidence, and when patients and families are confident that their providers are using evidence-based care, optimal outcomes are achieved (Melnyk & Fineout-Overholt, 2005). The Institute of Medicine (IOM) (2001) has designated evidence-based decision-making as an essential skill for health care. Patient outcomes have been shown to be 28 percent better when care is based on research, rather than on tradition (Melnyk & Fineout-Overholt, 2005).

Health care providers who use EBP report greater professional satisfaction than providers who base care on tradition or common practice (Melnyk, 2007). EBP can not only promote quality clinical care, but it also may reduce high nurse turnover rates, thereby possibly reducing nursing care costs (Melnyk, 2007). The IOM *Health Professions Education* report challenges nursing faculties and other health professions to produce clinical nurses who can implement EBP care as members of interdisciplinary teams.

> Nursing management during the early newborn period includes identification of risk factors, assessment, monitoring, intervention and postdischarge follow-up.

Eventually third-party payers may provide reimbursement only for health care practices proven effective by scientific evidence (Melnyk, 2007). Additionally, health care consumers are using the Web to find the latest treatment information on their health conditions. Informed consumers escalate the pressure on nurses and other health care providers to provide the most up-to-date practices and health-related information in patient care.

A gap exists between the publication of research evidence and its incorporation into practice. Professional organizations, such as the Association for Women's Health, Obstetric and Neonatal Nurses (AWHONN) and the National Association of Neonatal Nurses (NANN), are encouraging initiatives to narrow this gap and speed up mechanisms to translate research findings into clinical practice (Cronenwett, 2002; Melnyk, 2007).

Developmental care is a frame of reference on which to base all newborn care in the hospital and at home. It is individualized treatment based on diagnosis, gestational age and infant needs and capabilities. It often is associated with clinical bedside caregiving activities, such as positioning, handling, cobedding, environmental modifications and skin-to-skin contact. Developmental care identifies infant behavior as a means of communication that fosters infant-driven and relationship-building caregiving. It should be family-centered, with the realization that parents or other family or friends are the ultimate infant caregivers. The clinician's roles are to meet the medical needs of the infant and help the family and infant move to the next level of health, growth and development (Waitzman, 2007). The nurse and the infant's family are full partners in care. The partnership is based on the nurse's respect for the family's preferences, values and specific needs (Cronenwett et al., 2007).

High-risk infants are dependent on and vulnerable to their early environment. They may be cared for in a special nursery or neonatal intensive care unit (NICU) to maintain their physiologic function and to promote growth and development. Natural light, soothing colors, therapeutic sounds and family interaction can enhance newborn healing (Altimier, 2004). Changing traditional hospital policies and environment can produce an efficient, peaceful and satisfying setting for administering and receiving developmental infant care.

Cardiovascular and Pulmonary Adaptation

Successful transition to extrauterine life requires cardiopulmonary adaptation from placental to pulmonary gas exchange and from fetal to neonatal and adult circulation. Fetal lungs are largely nonfunctional, and the fetal liver is only partially functional due to placental oxygenation and metabolic activities. Placental circulation, which bypasses the heart, lungs and liver, provides the cardiac functions as the fetus grows. Consequently, these organs do not require large quantities of blood flow in utero. The route of fetal circulation, therefore, differs from neonatal and adult circulation. Table 1 identifies fetal blood flow characteristics.

Catecholamines that signal labor, along with the mother's hormones, help the fetus to mature and be ready for delivery. Although the labor process is mildly asphyxiating, most fetuses manage it well. Umbilical cord clamping stimulates peripheral and central chemoreceptors, causes tactile and thermal stimulation and

<table>
<tr><td colspan="1">Table 1. Anatomic Features of Fetal Blood Flow</td></tr>
<tr><td>

- The placenta is the exchange organ for oxygen and carbon dioxide and for nutrients and wastes.
- The ductus venosus permits most of the blood from the placenta to bypass the liver and enter the inferior vena cava. Forty-six percent of umbilical venous blood bypasses the lungs.
- The foramen ovale is the opening in the interatrial septum through which a portion of the blood flows from the right atrium directly to the left atrium.
- The patent ductus arteriosus (PDA) is a tubular shunt between the pulmonary artery and the descending aorta that allows blood to flow from the pulmonary artery to the aorta, bypassing the fetal lungs

</td></tr>
<tr><td>Lott, 2007</td></tr>
</table>

increases systemic blood pressure. These factors together usually are sufficient to make the neonate breathe vigorously.

At birth, the newborn undergoes dramatic and rapid changes in body systems to adapt to extrauterine existence. The most significant change is that the lungs become the primary organ of oxygenation. To facilitate the clearance of amniotic fluid from the neonate's lungs, the first few respirations must reach pressures of 20 cm H_2O to 40 cm H_2O to achieve a functional residual capacity (FRC). Initial respirations stimulate the release of surfactant from the lungs. Initial respirations, a decrease in PCO_2 and an increase in pH and PO_2 lower pulmonary vascular resistance.

When the umbilical cord is clamped, immediate circulatory changes occur because the placenta is no longer part of circulation. With the first breath and occlusion of the umbilical cord, the neonate's systemic resistance is elevated, causing a decrease in the amount of blood flow through the ductus arteriosus. Cord occlusion causes an increase in blood pressure and a corresponding stimulation of the aortic baroreceptors and the sympathetic nervous system. The onset of respirations and expansion of the lungs causes decreased pulmonary vascular resistance due to the direct effect of oxygen and carbon dioxide on the blood vessels (Lott, 2007).

Most of the right ventricular output flows through the lungs, increasing the blood flow from the lungs to the left atrium. This increase causes the pressure in the left atrium of the heart to increase. Increased pressure in the left atrium, combined with increased systemic vascular resistance, causes functional closure of the foramen ovale.

After birth, the umbilical vein and arteries are sealed and no longer transport blood. The ductus arteriosus normally closes within 15 hours to 24 hours after birth. This closure is caused by increased arterial oxygen content, primarily due to the onset of pulmonary respiration. Clamping the umbilical cord causes blood flow through the ductus venosus to cease; it is functionally closed by 1 week to 2 weeks after birth. The ductus arteriosus is anatomically sealed by constriction by 3 weeks to 4 weeks of age.

Because anatomic closure of the fetal pathways lags behind functional closure, the shunts may open and close intermittently before anatomic closure, resulting in transient functional murmurs. Pressure in the pulmonary artery remains high for several hours after birth. Blood flow direction through the ductus arteriosus reverses as pulmonary vascular resistance diminishes. Initially bidirectional, the flow becomes entirely left-to-right and is functionally insignificant by approximately 15 hours after birth. Functional murmurs do not cause any cardiovascular compromise and are not clinically significant.

Conditions that cause transient opening of fetal shunts, allowing unoxygenated blood to flow from the right side of the heart to the left, thereby bypassing the pulmonary circuit, produce transient cyanosis. Nurses should carefully evaluate and monitor any murmur or cyanosis in the neonate because they are signs of cardiovascular abnormalities (Lott, 2007).

Hypoxemia can cause a constricted ductus arteriosus to reopen and may re-establish increased pulmonary vascular resistance, leading to persistent pulmonary hypertension of the newborn. The ductus arteriosus responds to hypoxemia by opening, whereas the pulmonary arterioles respond by constricting (Lott, 2007; Morris, 2007b).

Fetal lungs secrete fetal lung fluid (FLF) throughout gestation. At term, FLF is 10 mL/kg to 25 mL/kg of body weight; this fluid must be expelled or absorbed at birth (Blackburn, 2007). As gestation progresses, the lungs become less secretory. Early theories of FLF removal emphasized the thoracic squeeze during vaginal birth, especially to explain retained FLF after cesarean birth. Later studies (Jain & Eaton, 2006) emphasized the importance of labor and concomitant catecholamine release as important stimuli for the lungs to stop secreting lung fluid. Neonates born via elective cesarean delivery have lower levels of catecholamines than neonates born vaginally or neonates subjected to a trial of labor but born via cesarean for reasons other than fetal distress (Blackburn, 2007; Jain & Eaton, 2006). Transient tachypnea of the newborn (TTN) is more common in infants born via elective cesarean who do not get the benefit of labor (Kenner & Lott, 2007).

Circulatory and lymphatic systems remove remaining fetal lung fluid via the circulatory and lymphatic systems as evidenced by distention of the interstitial spaces and lymphatic system during the first 5 hours to 6 hours of life and by an increase in pulmonary lymph flow (Blackburn, 2007). During this time, crackles may be auscultated across the newborn's lung fields.

Apgar Score

In 1952, Dr. Virginia Apgar devised a rapid scoring system to assess the clinical status of the newborn and the need for prompt intervention to establish breathing (Apgar, 1953). The Apgar score evaluates five physiologic signs (Table 2) at 1 minute and 5 minutes of life. Each sign is assigned a score of 0, 1 or 2, for a possible total score of 0 to 10. The Apgar score is a convenient shorthand for reporting newborn status and response to resuscitation (American Academy of Pediatrics [AAP] & American College of Obstetricians and Gynecologists [ACOG], 2007). However, nurses should recognize limitations of the Apgar score and educate families who may misunderstand its purpose. Table 3 identifies factors that can influence an Apgar score. The incidence of low Apgar scores is inversely related to birthweight. A low score is limited in predicting morbidity or mortality.

Component	Score		
	0	**1**	**2**
Heart rate (beats/minute)	Absent	Slow (<100)	>100
Respiration	Absent	Weak cry, hypoventilation	Good, strong cry
Muscle tone	Limp	Some flexion	Active motion
Reflex irritability	No response	Grimace	Cry or active withdrawal
Color	Blue or pale	Body pink, extremities blue	Completely pink

Table 2. Apgar Score

AAP, 1996. Reproduced with permission from *Pediatrics*, 98, 141-142. © 1996 by the AAP.

Table 3. Factors that Can Influence an Apgar Score

- Gestational age
- Congenital malformations
- Maternal medications
- Infection
- Brainstem dysfunction
- Hypoxia
- Hypovolemia
- Hypothermia

The Apgar score has been used inappropriately in term infants to predict specific neurologic outcome. Apgar scores are guidelines and do not dictate resuscitative actions. A delay in resuscitation to obtain an Apgar is not appropriate if an infant appears depressed (AAP & ACOG, 2007; AAP & AHA, 2006). However, an Apgar score that remains 0 beyond 10 minutes of age may be useful in determining whether additional resuscitative efforts are indicated.

The Apgar score should be assigned at 1 minute and 5 minutes of age during resuscitation; when the score is <7, additional scores should be obtained every 5 minutes for up to 20 minutes (AAP Committee on Fetus and Newborn & ACOG Committee on Obstetrical Practice, 2006). An Apgar score assigned during resuscitation is not equivalent to a score assigned to a spontaneously breathing infant because mechanical and drug interventions may be used (Lopriore, van Burk, Walther & Arnout, 2004).

Asphyxia

Two categories of asphyxia occur in the fetus and neonate. Fetal asphyxia (intrauterine asphyxia) is the reduction or cessation of placental gas exchange that occurs before or during delivery. Perinatal asphyxia is failure of the newborn to establish adequate alveolar ventilation at birth with subsequent hypoxemia and respiratory and metabolic acidosis (Blackburn, 2007). The diagnosis of asphyxia is used for litigation in cases of cerebral palsy and mental retardation.

The term perinatal asphyxia has been used inconsistently and inaccurately as a diagnosis. AAP and ACOG (2007) recommended using the term birth asphyxia to refer to the clinical situation of damaging academia, hypoxia and metabolic acidosis. Table 4 defines criteria for neurologic sequelae caused by perinatal asphyxia. Table 5 identifies effects of birth asphyxia.

Table 4. Criteria for Neurologic Sequelae Caused by Birth Asphyxia

• Profound metabolic or mixed acidemia (pH <7.00) on an umbilical artery sample
• Persistent low Apgar score of 0 to 3 for >5 minutes
• Evidence of neonatal neurologic sequelae (seizures, hypotonia, coma)
• Multisystem organ failure in the immediate neonatal period involving one or more of the following systems:
  – Cardiovascular
  – Gastrointestinal
  – Hematologic
  – Pulmonary
  – Renal

AAP & ACOG 2007

Table 5. Effects of Birth Asphyxia	
Neurologic effects	• Seizures • Abnormal respiratory patterns • Apnea • Respiratory arrest • Hyperalertness • Jitteriness • Posturing and movement disorders • Impaired suck, swallow, gag and feeding • Abnormal eye movements and pupillary responses • Hypotonia and lethargy • Bulging anterior fontanel (du Plessis, 2005)
Pulmonary effects	• Hypertension • Surfactant deficiency • Meconium aspiration syndrome
Renal effects	• Oliguria • Hematuria • Proteinuria • Renal failure • Renal vein thrombosis
Acute cardiovascular effects	• Tricuspid insufficiency • Myocardial necrosis • Cardiogenic shock/hypotension
Gastrointestinal effects	• Necrotizing enterocolitis (NEC) • Hepatic dysfunction
Hematologic effects	• Thrombocytopenia • Disseminated intravascular coagulopathy

Intrauterine asphyxia is the most frequent cause of acidosis in the neonate and brain injury in the full-term newborn (Kenner & Lott, 2007). There are three categories of obstetric risk factors for asphyxia: (1) altered placental gas exchange, (2) altered maternal perfusion of the placenta and (3) maternal hypoxemia (Blackburn, 2007). Birth asphyxia is related to birth trauma, failed initiation of respiration, respiratory distress syndrome (RDS) and apnea. The healthy term fetus or newborn can reduce overall oxygen consumption and protect vital organs, such as the brain and the heart, in response to hypoxemia and the threat of asphyxia.

When severe inadequate perfusion overwhelms the compensatory mechanisms, hypoxic-ischemic tissue damage results. If adequate oxygenation and perfusion are quickly restored, then injury is reversible. If not, then the goal is to prevent secondary insults or limit ongoing brain cell injury triggered by the initial insult (du Plessis, 2005).

Neurologic injury from birth asphyxia results from an inadequate oxygen supply to the brain. Oxygen supplies may be inadequate because of hypoxia, low amounts of oxygen in the blood or ischemia (low flow of blood to the nervous system). Hypoxia and ischemia typically are present during birth-asphyxial events. Hypoxic-ischemic encephalopathy (HIE) is a subtype of neonatal encephalopathy caused by limited oxygen and blood flow near the time of birth. HIE specifically describes central nervous system (CNS) findings associated with documented severe metabolic acidosis (Figueroa, Khabbaz & Quirk, 2005). Birth asphyxia with severe HIE can cause death. Researchers are studying whether hypothermia, with body cooling induced before 6 hours of age and continuing for 72 hours, reduces the incidence of morbidity and mortality associated with HIE (Shankaran et al., 2005).

Acute multisystem dysfunction and failure require intensive care and intervention. Therapy is geared toward ventilation support and perfusion and treatment of seizures. Neonatal seizures may occur secondary to intracranial hemorrhage, hypoglycemia, hypocalcemia, neurodevelopmental abnormalities and drug withdrawal (Kenner & Lott, 2007). Compared to controlled seizures, multiple or extended

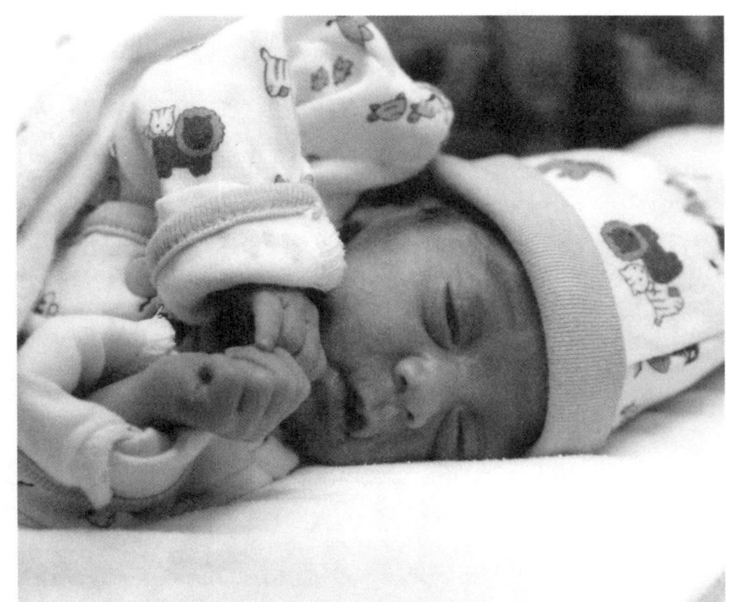

seizure activity is associated with significantly poorer prognosis (Kenner & Lott, 2007). If the infant survives the acute phase, long-term follow up is necessary to monitor CNS function for residual sequelae.

Delivery Management

Delivery management, including personnel, equipment, education and planning, is a vital aspect of perinatal services. Ten percent of all newborns require some form of assistance at birth, and 1 percent require extensive resuscitation (Wu & Carlo, 2002). Health care personnel who attend deliveries should be prepared to intervene appropriately.

Every birth should be attended by at least one person skilled in neonatal resuscitation whose sole responsibility is management of the newborn. Adequate history and identification of maternal and fetal risk factors can help nurses recognize neonates who may need resuscitation and plan for additional personnel to be available (Merrill & Ballard, 2005). Delivery rooms should be stocked at all times with resuscitation equipment. Per hospital policy, nurses should check equipment to ensure its working condition. Nurses also should check medication for sterile packaging and expiration dates.

Oxygen use in delivery varies from institution to institution. When a term infant is cyanotic or requires positive-pressure ventilation (PPV), NRP guidelines (AAP & AHA, 2006) recommend the use of 100 percent oxygen. If resuscitation is started with <100 percent oxygen, nurses should give supplemental oxygen up to 100 percent if there is no improvement within 90 seconds.

Resuscitation of an infant with an initial Apgar score of 0 is difficult. Discontinuation of resuscitation may be justified after 10 minutes of continuous and adequate resuscitation efforts if there are no signs of life (AAP & AHA, 2006; AHA, 2005). Infants who respond after 20 minutes of resuscitation show unacceptably high incidences of death or severe, irreversible neurologic damage.

Airway Assessment and Suctioning

Most term infants need little or no suctioning. If needed, suctioning may be done with a bulb syringe or a suction catheter. The nurse first suctions the mouth in case the infant gasps, and then the nose. The nose is suctioned because infants are obligatory nose breathers—they try to breathe through the nose after their initial cries. Suctioning with a catheter is performed gently. The nurse should pass the catheter 5 cm from the lips for 5 seconds, allowing for recovery time between suctioning. Vigorous suctioning and continued stimulation of the posterior portion of the pharynx can induce bradycardia.

Meconium

Meconium in the amniotic fluid complicates a small percentage of deliveries. AHA and NRP guidelines no longer recommend intrapartum (head delivered but not shoulders) oropharyngeal and nasopharyngeal suctioning because they do not reduce the incidence of meconium aspiration syndrome (AAP & AHA, 2006; Zaichkin, 2006). When a baby is born but not vigorous, endotracheal suctioning is required before the infant is dried or stimulated. An infant is classified as not vigorous if he has absent or depressed respirations, decreased muscle tone or a heart rate <100 beats per minute (AAP & AHA, 2006).

Effects of Anesthesia/Analgesia on the Neonate

Women often receive anesthesia and analgesia during labor for pain control. An analgesic diminishes pain sensation, thereby raising the pain threshold. An anesthetic may provide analgesia, and it may inhibit pain perception, thereby relaxing muscles. Most anesthesia and analgesia medications cross the placenta and enter the fetal circulation in a dose-dependent fashion (Mercer, Erickson-Owens, Graves & Haley, 2007). Providers should consider the effects on the fetus and newborn when deciding which drugs to use in labor.

Neurobehavioral effects of anesthetics on the neonate include CNS depression and neurobehavioral changes. When assessed on scales, such as the Neonatal Behavioral Assessment Scale (NBAS) or the Early Neonatal Neurobehavioral Scale (ENNS), infants of mothers who receive narcotic analgesia or epidural anesthesia perform less well on tests of muscle tone, alertness and motor skills than infants of mothers who do not receive anesthesia or analgesia; however, these effects are transient and resolve themselves within the first few days of life (Mercer, et al., 2007).

Assessment of Gestational Age

Before 1960, birthweight was the only criterion used to determine a newborn's maturity. Consequently, an infant whose birthweight was >2,500 g (5 lbs, 5 oz) was considered term. Newborn size, however, is affected by conditions that accelerate or retard fetal growth, resulting in discrepancies between growth and maturity. For example, in the case of maternal diabetes with maternal hyperglycemia, an infant may be born prematurely but larger than a term infant. In the case of uteroplacental insufficiency, an infant may be born at term but small. Accurate assessment of gestational age incorporates size and maturity, facilitating identification of infants at risk, anticipation of clinical problems and planning of care.

Estimating Gestational Age

Providers use various methods to assess gestational age: the mother's menstrual history, prenatal ultrasonography, evaluation of obstetric parameters and postnatal maturational examinations. These methods are highly accurate and pose little or no risk to the infant. The basis of these methods is that fetal development normally proceeds in an organized, predictable manner. At a given gestational age, infants generally have many characteristics in common (Kenner & Lott, 2007).

Mother's Menstrual History

The best method of measurement is an exact menstrual history, which should be obtained as early as possible. Seventy-five percent to 85 percent of women accurately recall the onset date of their last menstrual period (LMP) (Kenner & Lott, 2007). Reasons for miscalculation include irregular menses, medically induced ovulation and postconception bleeding. Expected accuracy and reliability of dating based on the LMP is ±14.6 days, a total range of 4 weeks.

Prenatal Ultrasonography

One method for measuring gestational age is the prenatal ultrasound examination. Measurement of the crown-rump length is precise when performed early in gestation (6 weeks to 18 weeks). It allows for the most accurate assessment of gestational age within a range of +1 week. It decreases in certainty to +3 weeks from 29 weeks to term. As gestation progresses, fetal ultrasound measurements may be unavoidably inaccurate because the fetus is less visible by ultrasound as it descends into the birth canal. Late-trimester ultrasound results are less dependable than results obtained earlier in pregnancy.

Ultrasound is a noninvasive technology that providers often offer in the first trimester of pregnancy. However, it should be reserved for medical indications. Fetal magnetic resonance imaging (MRI) also can be used and appears to have little risk of radiation exposure; however more studies are needed to examine its use during pregnancy (AAP & ACOG, 2007).

Evaluating Obstetric Parameters

Providers use various obstetric milestones to estimate gestational age. At about 20 weeks of pregnancy, the first auscultation of fetal heart tones may be heard by fetoscope. Providers can measure fundal height, which is directly related to the weight of the fetus and duration of pregnancy. Also useful is the mother's report of quickening, which occurs around 18 weeks in primigravid women and somewhat earlier in multigravid women.

Postnatal Maturational Examinations

Another method of assessing gestational age is the postnatal maturational examination. After delivery, the infant's gestational age is estimated by assessing physical, neurologic and neuromuscular development. Several screening tools are available.

A variety of intrauterine experiences may influence fetal maturation. Stressful fetal experiences may increase pulmonary and neuromuscular rates of maturation, whereas physical maturation may be slowed or not affected. Events that accelerate fetal maturation may adversely affect fetal growth, and events that accelerate fetal growth may delay maturation.

The most important component of the postnatal maturational examination is the clinical observer. The more experienced the examiner, the more reliable and valid the data.

Dubowitz Assessment of Gestational Age

In 1970, Dubowitz, Dubowitz and Goldberg developed the Dubowitz Assessment of Gestational Age. In this assessment, neurologic response criteria are based on expected progression of neuromuscular maturation, which consists of flexor tone replacing extensor tone in a caudocephalad (tail-to-head) progression. The assessment looks at neurologic and external physical signs (Table 6). The provider scores each area and correlates the scores with weeks of gestation. Providers should perform this examination within the first 5 days of life because physical characteristics may start to change after this time.

Table 6. Dubowitz Assessment of Gestational Age	
External physical signs	• Skin characteristics • Plantar creases • Nipple and breast development • Ear development and formation • Appearance of the genitalia
Neurologic signs	• Resting posture • Square window • Ankle dorsiflexion • Arm recoil • Leg recoil • Popliteal angle • Heel-to-ear • Scarf sign • Head lag • Ventral suspension

Dubowitz, Dubowitz & Goldberg, 1970

Lubchenco Scale

In 1972, Lubchenco and colleagues developed a new scale for clinical estimation of gestational age. The Lubchenco scale is used during the first hours of life. Assessment requires little or no handling of the newborn. When a discrepancy occurs between the assessment and gestational age based on the mother's menstrual history, a neurological examination can be performed at 24 hours of age when the infant is more stable. The initial examination may provide information beyond gestational age, such as evidence of intrauterine growth restriction (IUGR).

New Ballard Maturational Exam

In 1979, Ballard, Novak and Driver developed the New Ballard Maturational Exam to assess gestational age. It was derived from the Newborn Maturity Rating, a simplified version of the Dubowitz tool. The exam has been refined and expanded to achieve greater accuracy and to include extremely premature infants (Ballard et al., 1991). The New Ballard eliminates a neurological assessment, which requires active muscle tone and can be difficult to assess in ill infants. The exam should occur within the first 48 hours of life (Tappero & Honeyfield, 2003).

The exam is based on six neuromuscular and six physical criteria (Figure 1). A score of -1 to 5 is assigned to each criterion. If a sign falls between the scoring options, a half score may be assigned. After assessing and scoring all 12 items, a total score is calculated and compared to the maturity rating table to estimate the infant's gestational age. For example, a score of 37 corresponds to a gestational age between 38 weeks and 40 weeks.

Figure 1. Maturational Assessment of Gestational Age (New Ballard Score)

Neuromuscular Maturity

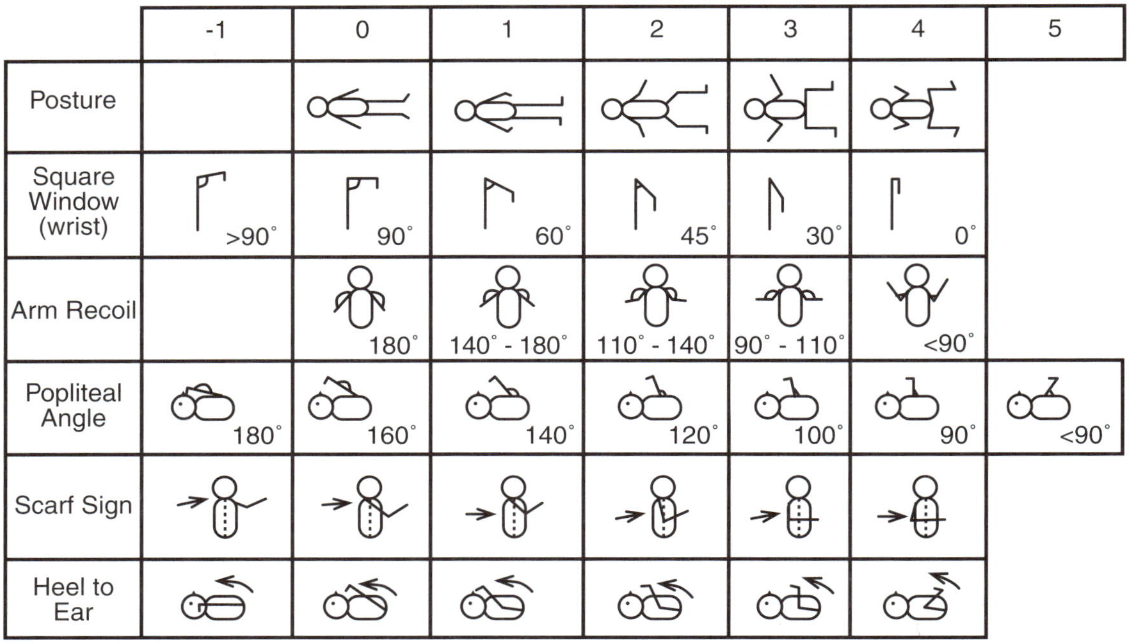

	-1	0	1	2	3	4	5
Posture							
Square Window (wrist)	>90°	90°	60°	45°	30°	0°	
Arm Recoil		180°	140° - 180°	110° - 140°	90° - 110°	<90°	
Popliteal Angle	180°	160°	140°	120°	100°	90°	<90°
Scarf Sign							
Heel to Ear							

Physical Maturity

Skin	sticky iriable transparent	gelatinous red, translucent	smooth pink visible veins	superficial peeling &/or rash few veins	cracking pale areas rare veins	parchment deep cracking no vessels	leathery cracked wrinkled
Lanugo	none	sparse	abundant	thinning	bald areas	mostly bald	
Plantar Surface	heel-toe 40-50 mm:-1 < 40 mm:-2	>50mm no crease	faint red marks	anterior transverse crease only	creases ant. 2/3	creases over entire sole	
Breast	imperceptible	barely perceptible	flat areola no bud	slipped areola 1-2mm bud	raised areola 3-4mm bud	full areola 5-10mm bud	
Eye/Ear	lids fused loosely:-1 tightly:-2	lids open pinna flat stays folded	sl. curved pinna; soft; slow recoil	well-curved pinna: soft but ready recoil	formed & firm instant recoil	thick cartillage ear stiff	
Genitals male	scrotum flat, smooth	scrotum empty faint rugae	testes in upper canal rare rugae	testes descending few rugae	testes down good rugae	testes pendulous deep rugae	
Genitals female	clitoris prominent labia flat	prominent clitoris small labia minora	prominent clitoris enlarging minora	majora & minora equally prominent	majora large minora small	majora cover clitoris & minora	

Maturity Rating

score	weeks
-10	20
-5	22
-0	24
5	26
10	28
15	30
20	32
25	34
30	36
35	38
40	40
45	42
50	44

Ballard, Khoury, Wedig, Wang, Eilers-Walsman & Lipp, 1991. Reprinted with permission from Elsevier.

Infant Classification and Growth Assessment

After assessing gestational age, the provider plots the infant's length, weight and occipital-frontal head circumference (OFC) on intrauterine growth charts (Figure 2). Growth curves show measures of intrauterine growth in percentiles for each week of gestation. Table 7 identifies infant classification by percentile. Using the growth curve, a newborn weighing 3,600 gm at 40 weeks is term appropriate for gestational age (AGA), but an infant weighing 3,600 gm at 37 weeks is term large for gestational age (LGA). Small for gestational age (SGA), LGA, premature and postmature infants may be at risk for postnatal morbidity or mortality complications and should be closely observed in the nursery (Kenner & Lott, 2007). AGA term newborns have lower mortality and morbidity rates than SGA and LGA term newborns (Figure 3).

Several intrauterine growth curves have been developed for specific populations. Two commonly used curves are the Oregon and Colorado curves. The Oregon curves are normed on 40,000 live, singleton infants born at sea level between 1959 and 1966 to Caucasian women who were cared for by private physicians (Babson, Behrman & Lessel, 1970). The Colorado curves are based on 4,700 newborns born to medically indigent White (55 percent), Hispanic (30 percent) and Black (15 percent) mothers at an altitude of 5,280 feet (Lubchenco, Searls & Brazie, 1972). The Oregon curves assess weight only.

LGA

Table 8 identifies complications, increased risks and birth injuries associated with LGA. Genetically large newborns do not have increased risks related to pathophysiologic processes. Infants of diabetic mothers with poor serum glucose control receive excess glucose via the placenta and respond with hyperinsulinemia. Consequently, these infants are prone to excess body fat and glycogen stores, increased muscle mass and organomegaly, especially heart and liver. Infants with cephalohematoma are at increased risk for hyperbilirubinemia. Screening blood glucose levels is an important assessment for these infants.

SGA

Table 9 identifies maternal and fetal factors and increased fetal risks associated with SGA. Conditions associated with SGA place newborns at greater risk for mortality than AGA or LGA infants.

Providers often use the terms SGA and IUGR synonymously. IUGR denotes a pathophysiologic process that results in fetal growth restriction, whereas SGA refers to infants who fall below the tenth percentile on a growth curve. IUGR infants are often SGA; however, a fetus who has stopped growing in utero and is delivered before falling below the tenth percentile is correctly termed IUGR, not SGA.

AGA term newborns have lower mortality and morbidity rates than SGA and LGA term newborns.

Figure 2. Growth Chart

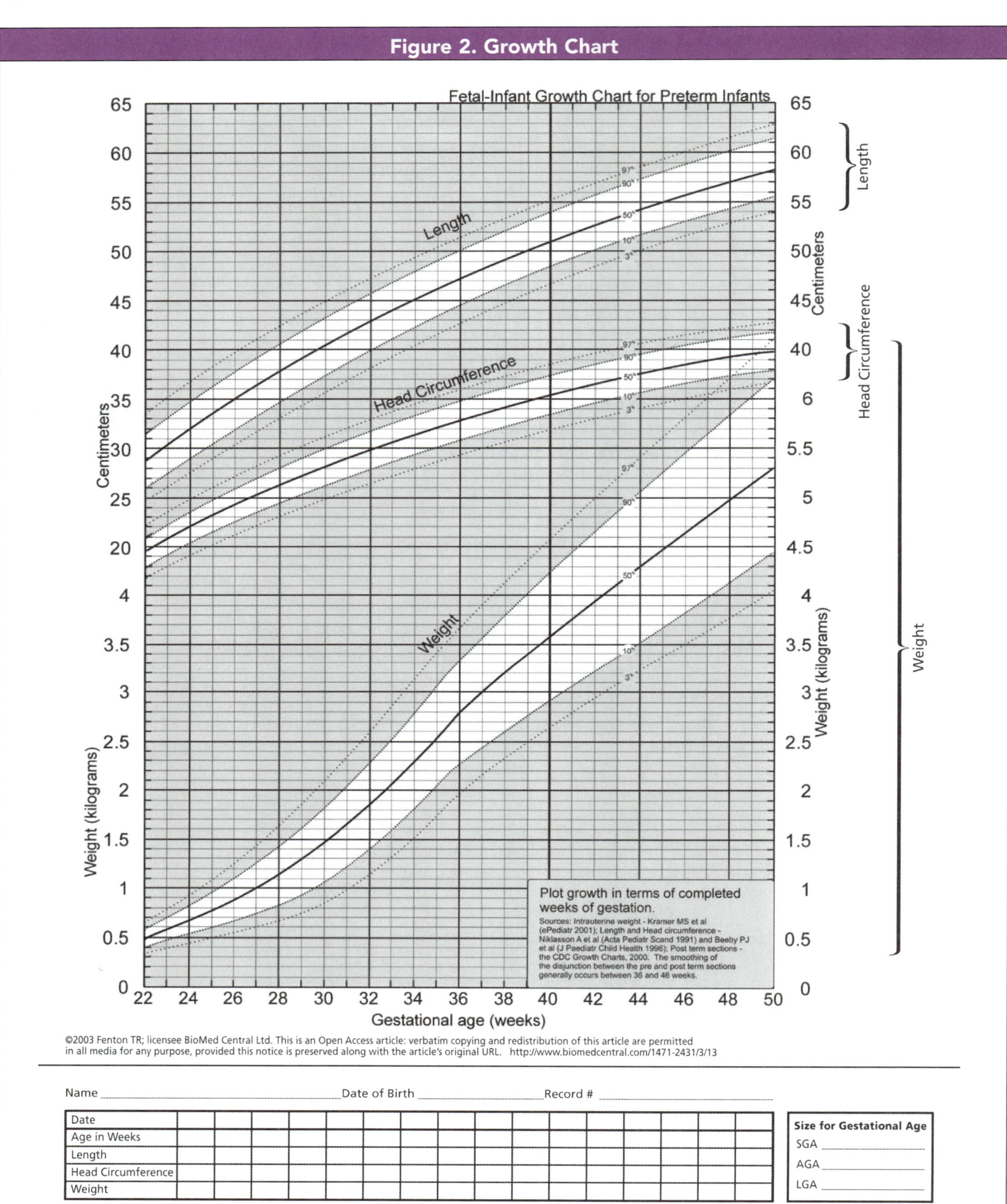

©2003 Fenton TR; licensee BioMed Central Ltd. This is an Open Access article: verbatim copying and redistribution of this article are permitted in all media for any purpose, provided this notice is preserved along with the article's original URL. http://www.biomedcentral.com/1471-2431/3/13

This chart can be used for preterm and term infants.

Table 7. Infant Classification by Growth Assessment

Term	Percentile
Large for gestational age (LGA)	Above the 90th percentile
Appropriate for gestational age (AGA)	Between the tenth and 90th percentiles
Small for gestational age (SGA)	Below the tenth percentile

Figure 3. Morbidity Table. Deviations of Intrauterine Growth: Neonatal Morbidity by Birthweight and Gestational Age

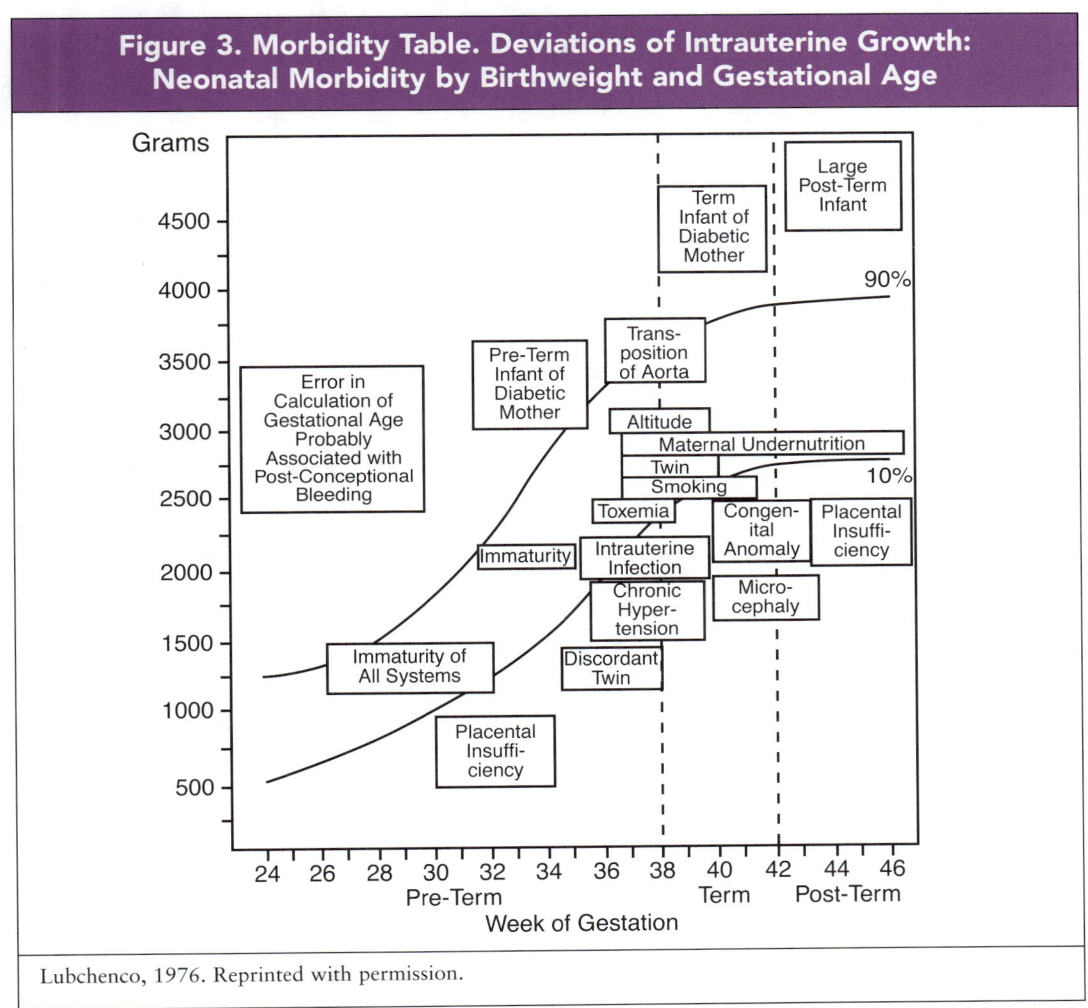

Lubchenco, 1976. Reprinted with permission.

Table 8. Factors and Complications Associated with LGA	
Maternal complications	• Post-term gestation • Maternal diabetes with hyperglycemia • Maternal obesity • Genetically large babies (of large parents) • Transposition of the great vessels • Beckwith-Wiedemann syndrome • Erythroblastosis fetalis
Infant risks	• Prolonged labor • Shoulder dystocia • Birth injury • Postnatal respiratory depression from difficult deliveries • Hypoglycemia (secondary to fetal hyperinsulinism) (Blackburn, 2007)
Birth injuries	• Bruising • Cephalohematomas • Facial nerve palsy • Fractured clavicle • Brachial plexus injury

Table 9. Factors and Complications Associated with SGA	

Complications	**Maternal**
	• Poor maternal weight gain during pregnancy
	• Multiparity
	• Chronic maternal disease
	• Multiple gestation
	• Uteroplacental insufficiency
	  – Heart disease
	  – Renal disease
	  – Hypertension
	  – Preeclampsia
	  – Post-term pregnancy
	  – Sickle cell disease
	  – Smoking
	
	Fetal
	• Chromosomal abnormalities
	• Skeletal system malformations
	• Congenital infections, such as cytomegalovirus (CMV) or rubella

Newborn risks	• Hypoglycemia • Secondary to diminished glycogen stores • Hypothermia due to decreased subcutaneous tissue • Hypoxia during labor and delivery, particularly when growth retardation results from chronic uteroplacental insufficiency • Polycythemia • Hyperbilirubinemia

Physical Assessment

Nurses should systematically conduct a newborn's physical assessment. The examination should occur within the first 24 hours of life after transition is complete (Verklan & Walden, 2004). Table 10 identifies information with which the nurse should be familiar before the examination.

The examination area should be well lit, warm and free of drafts to prevent loss of body heat. A radiant warmer may be used. The infant should be in a quiet state. The nurse observes the infant for spontaneous motor activity, bilateral symmetry of active movements, resistance to passive range of motion and the ability to calm himself. The healthy term infant displays a flexed posture, indicating good muscle tone. Spontaneous activity should be symmetrical with flexion and extension of the arms and legs.

Table 10. Information to Review Before a Newborn Physical Assessment
• Maternal and paternal medical histories • The course of pregnancy, labor and delivery • The birth history • Condition of the infant at birth • Apgar scores • Resuscitative measures • Laboratory values • Treatments
Kenner & Lott, 2007

Table 11 lists abnormal findings in a physical examination. These findings require further evaluation and follow-up. The neonatal assessment provides the base from which problems are identified and interventions are planned and implemented. It is a continuing process during infant care.

Table 11. Newborn Physical Examination: Abnormal Findings
• Asymmetrical movements • Floppy or rigid posture • Weak movements • High-pitched cry • Prolonged tremors • Inability to complete a full range of motion

Weight and Length

The nurse weighs the quiet infant without clothing or diaper. Weight can be falsely increased by a significant amount of infant motion. Weight should be recorded in pounds/ounces and in grams.

An AGA term infant weighs 2,500 g to 4,000 g; it is acceptable for infants to lose up to 10 percent of their birthweight in the first week of life (Kenner & Lott, 2007). However, with adequate hydration and feeding, this loss often does not occur. Infants should return to their birthweight within the first 2 weeks of life. Generally infants double their birthweight by 4 months to 5 months of age (Tappero & Honeyfield, 2003).

Nurses use a crown-to-heel measurement for infant length. The infant should be supine with the legs extended and the head flat. The nurse draws a line on the bed at the infant's head and another at the heels. The distance between these two points is the infant's length. The term infant's length averages 45 cm to 55 cm (Kenner & Lott, 2007). Because of head molding and incomplete extension of the knees, direct measurement of the infant is difficult.

Nurses should systematically conduct a newborn's physical assessment. The examination should occur within the first 24 hours of life after transition is complete.

Vital Signs

The healthy infant has a respiratory rate between 40 and 60 breaths per minute (Kenner & Lott, 2007). It is acceptable for the rate to be irregular. Respirations should be easy and unlabored. Respiratory rates may vary, but persistent tachypnea (respiratory rate >60 breaths per minute) may indicate underlying lung conditions, such as transient tachypnea of the newborn, RDS, meconium aspiration or pneumonia (Tappero & Honeyfield, 2003). On auscultation, breath sounds should be clear.

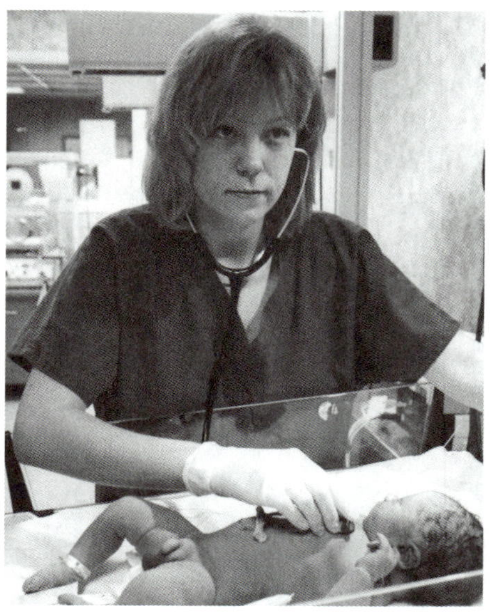

Heart rate should range from 120 to 160 beats per minute (Kenner & Lott, 2007). Variation in this rate is a positive sign that the infant has the ability to react to his environment.

Blood pressure ranges are related to gestational and chronologic ages (Kenner & Lott, 2007). Table 12 shows infant blood pressure values. The nurse measures blood pressure while the infant is quiet.

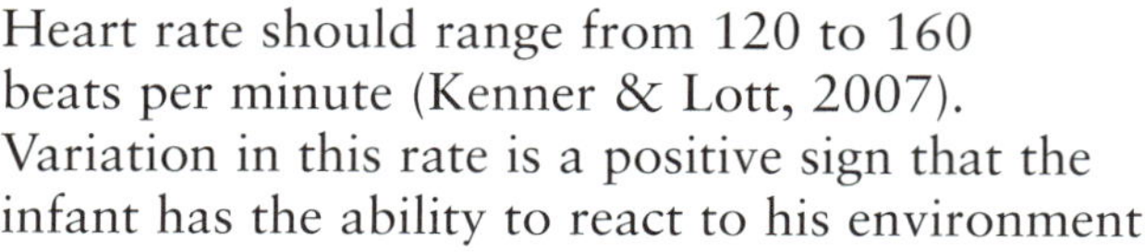

Table 12. Blood Pressure Values According to Site and Age				
Site	**Age**	**Blood Pressure (mm Hg)**		
		Systolic	Diastolic	Mean
Right arm	<36 hours old	62.6 ± 6.9	38.9 ± 5.7	48 ± 6.2
	>36 hours old	68.4 ± 8.8*	43.5 ± 6.2*	53 ± 7.3
	Total	64.7 ± 8.1	40.6 ± 6.2	49.8
Calf	<36 hours old	61.9 ± 7	39.6 ± 5.3	47.6 ± 6
	>36 hours old	66.8 ± 10.1*	42.5 ± 7.3*	51.5 ± 9*
	Total	63.6 ± 8.6	40.6 ± 6.3	49 ± 7.5

Values were obtained by blood pressure cuff measurement in 219 healthy term infants, 140 <36 hours old and 79 >36 hours old. Values are given as means ± standard deviation.

*Significantly different from values in infants <36 hours old (p <0.05).

Hegyi, et al., 1994. Reprinted with permission.

Skin

Table 13 lists the components of the initial skin assessment. The skin should be soft, smooth and opaque. Darker-skinned infants may be harder to assess for color, but the mucous membranes should be pink. The infant is undressed for a skin assessment (Brown, 2007).

The term infant is covered by vernix caseosa, a greasy or waxy, whitish or yellowish substance that appears early in the third trimester and begins to diminish at term. Vernix caseosa protects fetal skin in the aqueous environment against fluid loss and bacterial invasion. The term infant has subcutaneous fat that helps prevent heat loss. The nurse may note meconium staining in the creases of the skin, the umbilicus and the nails; it is most common in the postmature infant (Tappero & Honeyfield, 2003).

Variation from regular skin color may occur. Acrocyanosis is common and may occur in the transition period. The lips are generally pink, but the hands and feet are bluish. The blue color is caused by sluggish circulation and poor peripheral perfusion resulting from venous stress or cold stress. Once the infant is warmed, the color should improve. General cyanosis is not normal; it may be present with cardiac or respiratory dysfunction. The infant should be evaluated for hypoxia.

Table 13. Initial Skin Assessment
• General color
• Consistency (smooth, peeling)
• Opacity
• Thickness
• Hair distribution
• Staining
• Epidermal consistency
• Obvious markings, moles or rashes

Jaundice is a yellowish color of the skin, mucous membranes and sclera resulting from elevated levels of unconjugated bilirubin. Jaundice is abnormal in infants <24 hours old and may indicate Rh incompatibility, sepsis or TORCH (toxoplasmosis, other viruses, rubella, cytomegalovirus and herpes simplex virus) infections. Jaundice can be noted by applying pressure to the skin and noting the yellowish color.

Mottling of the skin occurs in response to cold or other stressful stimuli. It is caused by dilation of capillaries. It is most obvious on the extremities but may occur on the trunk. Mottling should improve when the infant is warmed. If it does not improve, the nurse evaluates the infant for other conditions, such as cardiovascular hypertension.

Some infants may be pale. Paleness is caused by decreased circulating hemoglobin or intense cutaneous vasoconstriction and requires further evaluation.

Plethora is the ruddy, purplish color caused by increased amounts of circulating, unsaturated hemoglobin. Ruddy at birth generally has a red undertone; however, plethora has a purple undertone. Plethora requires further evaluation.

Infants may exhibit benign rashes that require assessment. Milia are tiny, sebaceous, inclusion cysts, usually seen on the chin, nose, forehead and cheeks. They are whitish, pinhead-sized papules. When appearing in the mouth, they are called Epstein pearls. No erythema is seen. They are benign findings that typically resolve within a few weeks of life.

Erythema toxic appears as white or yellowish papules on a red macular base. It may involve any part of the body but is usually found on the face, trunk or proximal extremities. It is common, occurring in 70 percent of term neonates; it peaks at 24 to 48 hours of age and recedes within a few days (Tappero & Honeyfield, 2003).

Pustular melanosis may appear at birth on any body area. They are initially small (2 mm) vesicopustules on the face, neck and submental area. The vesicles eventually rupture to show a hyperpigmented macule surrounded by a fine, scaly skin ring. They are more common in African-Americans than in other ethnic groups (Kenner & Lott, 2007).

Petechiae are blue-black pinpoint macules that cannot be blanched. These lesions generally are related to birth trauma and usually fade by the third to fourth day of life. Further evaluation is warranted if petechiae are widespread (Brown, 2007).

Ecchymosis appears as a large area of subcutaneous hemorrhage. The nurse may observe it on the presenting part in breech or traumatic deliveries. Ecchymosis results from trauma to underlying blood vessels and may result in early jaundice.

Forcep or vacuum-extraction marks may be seen over the face, head or presenting part. These marks are usually benign. If they are located on the face, the nurse observes the infant for facial nerve paralysis.

Sucking blisters may appear on the lips where the fetus has been sucking on skin in utero. These are benign findings that should resolve without intervention.

Several vascular anomalies may occur, including macular hemangioma, also known as a stork bite. It is commonly found on the occipital area, eyelids and glabella. These lesions usually have indistinct borders, are salmon-pink in color and easily blanched, and resolve within the first year of life. Pigmented birthmarks are lesions that are brown-black to blue in color. Vascular variations also are birthmarks, but they generally are red in color.

A port wine stain (nevus flammeus) usually is visible at birth. It does not blanch with pressure and does not disappear with time. It is sharply delineated, and the color is purple to red in light-skinned infants, but jet black in dark-skinned infants. If it is found over the trigeminal area of the face, it may be associated with an angiomatous malformation (Sturge-Weber syndrome) and requires further evaluation (Kenner & Lott, 2007).

Strawberry hemangiomas are bright red, vascular tumors with sharply demarcated margins. They are somewhat compressible and blanch with pressure to reveal underlying pigmentation. They are most commonly found on the face. Seventy percent of tumors spontaneously regress by age 7; treatment usually is unnecessary (Brown, 2007).

A cavernous hemangioma has less distinct margins but gives a reddish-blue color to overlying tissue. It usually increases in size after birth. It may be found anywhere on the body and may cause thrombocytopenia or hypertrophy of bone and soft structures of the extremities (Kenner & Lott, 2007). Most of these lesions regress with age, but some may require steroid therapy and in, severe cases, surgery.

Mongolian spots are large, dark blue or purple bruise-like macular spots. These lesions usually are located over the sacrum, buttocks, flanks or shoulders and disappear by 4 years of age. They are more common in infants with darker skin tones.

Café au lait spots are tan or brown macules or patches. They are usually <3 cm in diameter. They are not significant unless they are large (4 cm to 6 cm) or there are more than six spots. Having six or more café au lait spots may be linked with a genetic neurologic condition called neurofibromatosis. In this condition, the spots develop into tumors that attach to nerves and eventually affect bone and skin.

The harlequin sign is a vascular phenomenon represented by a distinct midline demarcation in side-lying infants. The dependent half is deep red, and the upper half is pale. This is a benign finding that lasts a few seconds to 30 minutes. If it is recurring or persistent, the nurse may consider a cardiac defect (Kenner & Lott, 2007).

Head

The nurse notes overall symmetry when examining the head. Head shape is affected partially by presentation and type of delivery. Infants born by cesarean section often have a rounded head, whereas those born by vaginal delivery in the vertex position may have a more irregularly shaped head. This irregular shape may last for a few days. Some congenital abnormalities (hydrocephalus) also may cause an abnormal head shape.

Nurses measure the head circumference from the most prominent part of the occipital area to the forehead above the eyebrows, avoiding the ears. The average head circumference in a term infant is 35 cm; the customary range is 31 cm to 38 cm (Kenner & Lott, 2007). As a general rule, the head circumference in centimeters is equal to one-half the length in centimeters plus 10 (Tappero & Honeyfield, 2003).

Microcephaly means having an unusually small head. It is associated with a number of congenital syndromes and underdevelopment of the brain. Hydrocephalus is a large head size associated with blocked cerebrospinal fluid circulation or with overproduction of cerebrospinal fluid (Kenner & Lott, 2007).

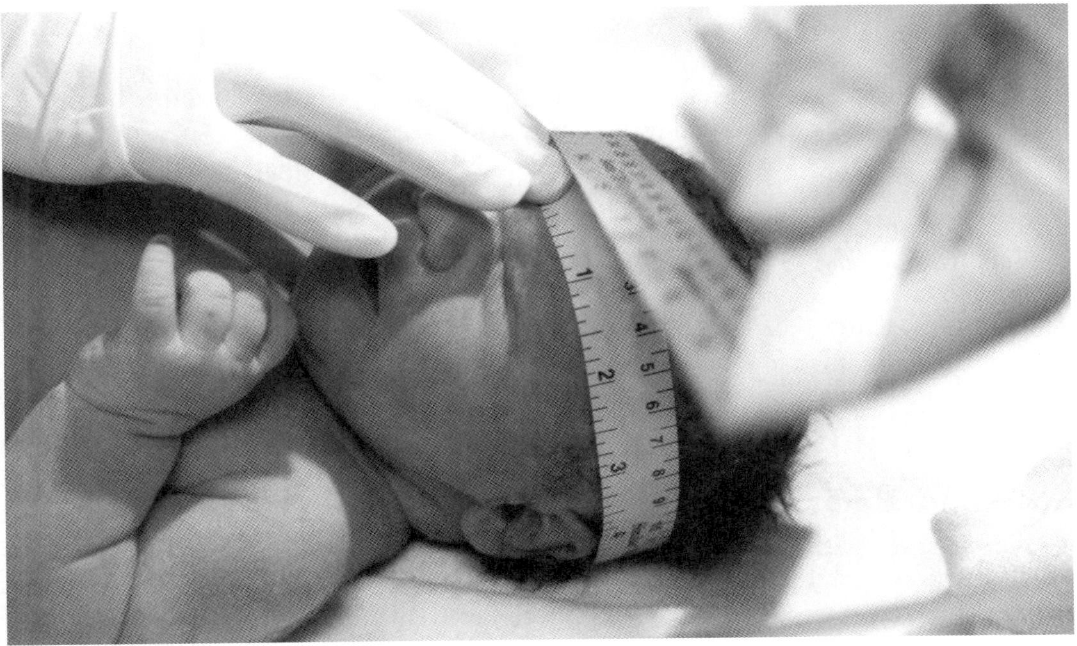

The presence of molding, caused by pressure from a vaginal delivery or edema, may alter the head circumference. The nurse repeats measure after this condition subsides. Skull sutures move freely and may overlap as a result of molding. If a large amount of molding is present, the nurse may need to re-evaluate the sutures after the molding has resolved.

The nurse examines the major bones of the head, sutures and the fontanels. The head is palpated to assess the firmness of bone and the size and configuration of fontanels and sutures, and to detect swelling, masses or bony defects (Kenner & Lott, 2007). The main sutures to be evaluated include the coronal, which separates the frontal from the parietal bones; the sagittal, which runs longitudinally in the midline between the two parietal bones; the lambdoidal, which extends posterolaterally from the posterior fontanel and separates the occipital from the parietal bones; and the squamous, which separates parietal from temporal bones. Premature close of sutures may result in an abnormal head shape (Tappero & Honeyfield, 2003).

The infant has as many as six palpable fontanels at birth; the two most important are the anterior and posterior fontanels. The anterior fontanel is a diamond-shaped, soft area at the junction of the coronal and sagittal sutures. In the term infant, its widest point is 2 cm to 3 cm. It closes during the first 18 months of life (Kenner & Lott, 2007). The posterior fontanel is triangular and located between the sagittal and lambdoidal sutures. It is 1 cm to 2 cm wide and may close during the last 2 months of gestation or in the first 2 months after birth. The fontanels are soft and flat. Full, tense or bulging fontanels may indicate increased intracranial pressure. "Sunken" fontanels indicate severe dehydration. These conditions require further evaluation (Brown, 2007).

Caput succedaneum may be present after delivery. This phenomenon is an edema of the superficial scalp tissue that extends across suture lines. It is the most common form of trauma occurring to the head (Kenner & Lott, 2007). It is most pronounced immediately after birth and subsides within 2 days to 3 days. It is caused by pressure on the head when the infant is in the vertex position. It is not clinically significant.

Cephalohematoma is a collection of blood between the periosteum and cranial bone. It has clearly demarcated edges confined by suture lines. It may form during labor and increase in size during the first 24 to 48 hours of life. Cephalohematomas usually resolve completely but may persist. Reabsorption may take 2 weeks to 3 weeks or longer (Kenner & Lott, 2007). A cephalohematoma may result in hyperbilirubinemia.

The nurse evaluates hair for color, length, continuity, texture and quantity. Term neonates usually have fine hair with identifiable individual hair strands. Patches of white hair may be benign, but a white forelock may be associated with deafness or mental retardation.

Face and Neck

The nurse assesses the face for shape, symmetry, bruising and dysmorphic features. Facial features should be proportional and symmetric. The nurse evaluates gag, sucking and rooting reflexes and checks facial movements for symmetry during crying and the neck for length, masses, webbing, mobility and the relationship of neck to body. Usually, the infant's neck is short. The presence of redundant skin at the posterolateral part is called web neck. Web neck may be associated with conditions such as Turner's syndrome and requires further evaluation. The nurse palpates the clavicles for fractures. The clavicles should be intact without swelling or crepitus.

Ears

The nurse examines the ears for position, shape, size and pits or tags. Ears should be positioned so the pinna aligns with the inner canthus of the eye. Asymmetry or irregular shape, size or position may be associated with congenital anomalies. Skin tags may be associated with renal anomalies. The term infant has cartilage throughout the helix of the ear, creating instant recoil of the ear when it is folded. The ear canal of the newborn infant is usually full of vernix, amniotic debris and blood; therefore, it is not always helpful to view the ear with an otoscope. This condition clears in approximately 60 percent of term infants by 1 week of age (Kenner & Lott, 2007). To assess the infant's hearing, the provider observes the infant's response to loud noises. The Centers for Disease Control and Prevention (CDC) (2007) recommends that all babies be screened for hearing impairment before 1 month of age, preferably before discharge from the hospital.

Eyes

The nurse examines the eyes for shape, position, size, movement, appearance of pupils, red reflex, hemorrhage or conjunctivitis. If abnormalities of the external eye are present, the nurse looks for other malformations. The sclera of the term infant is white. Very blue sclera is an abnormal finding that indicates a connective tissue disorder.

Tear formation does not occur until 2 months to 3 months of age. Because the nasolacrimal duct is not fully patent until 5 months to 7 months, even drainage in both eyes is common. Unless the drainage is accompanied by redness or swelling, it may be treated by lacrimal massage and gentle cleansing with water and a cotton ball (Tappero & Honeyfield, 2003).

The iris is incompletely pigmented for the first 6 months of life. Permanent eye color is not established for several months, but darker races may show permanent pigmentation in the first week of life. In general, the cornea appears shiny and glassy. The infant's lens transmits a clear red color called red reflex. Red reflex is achieved by holding a bright light 6 inches to 8 inches from the infant's eye to inspect the lens for cataracts. The pupils should be round and equal in diameter and should constrict equally in response to light—pupils equal and reactive to light (PERL) (Kenner & Lott, 2007).

Nose

The nurse assesses the nose for patency of nares, shape and symmetry, skin lesions and signs of trauma. The infant's nose generally is midline, symmetrical and flat. The nasal mucosa is pink and slightly moist. Secretions are thin, clear and scant. The nurse assesses patency by applying gentle pressure and occluding the opposite naris. The nurse checks for nasal flaring, which is abnormal and may indicate respiratory distress. Infants are obligate nose breathers, so if bilateral choanal atresia (obstruction of the posterior nasal passages) occurs, the infant is cyanotic at rest and pink when crying and breathing through the mouth (Tappero & Honeyfield, 2003).

Mouth

The examination of the mouth includes inspection and palpation of the lips, gums, tongue and palate. The nurse evaluates the mouth for size, shape, color and the presence of abnormal structures and masses. The mouth assessment may occur toward the end of the examination because it may upset the infant. Generally, the mouth is midline and symmetrical in shape and movement. Mucous membranes are pink and moist, and oral secretions are thin and clear (Kenner & Lott, 2007).

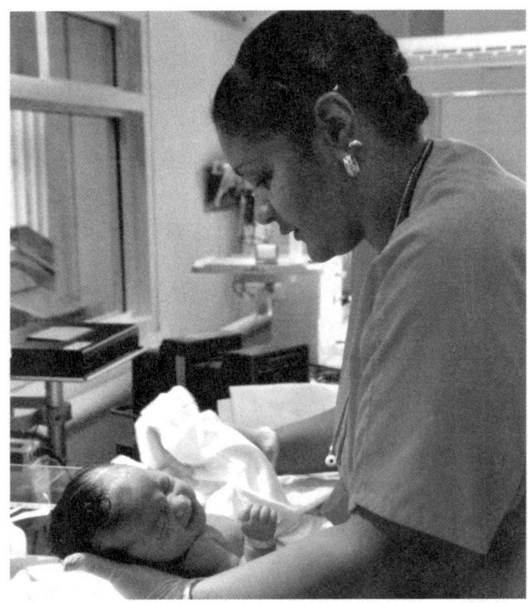

The nurse assesses the infant for cleft lip or palate. Cleft lip is a lateral defect that may occur alone or together with a cleft palate. The hard and soft palates should be examined for a cleft.

Thrush may be present in the mouth; it is identified as white patches that are difficult to remove. (White patches that are easily removed are caused from milk intake.) Thrush is a candidal infection that can be transmitted during the birth process. Epstein's pearls also may be present.

Natal teeth may be present and are usually seen in the lower incisor region. Typically, they are malformed and loose and should be removed.

An excess amount of saliva may indicate a tracheoesophageal fistula or esophageal atresia. The nurse should assess strength and coordination of the swallow reflex at every feeding. If there is concern about patency of the esophagus, the nurse inserts an orogastric tube (Tappero & Honeyfield, 2003). The infant's cry is assessed for quality, strength, pitch, hoarseness and stridor. The nurse also checks the infant's rooting and sucking reflexes (Brown, 2007).

Thorax and Cardiovascular System

The nurse assesses the infant's chest for size, symmetry, musculature, bony structure, number and location of nipples, and ease of respiration. The healthy newborn's chest appears round and symmetrical in shape and movement. The average chest circumference of a term infant is 33 ± 3 cm; it usually is 2 cm smaller than the head circumference (Kenner & Lott, 2007).

Two nipples are present in equal alignment. Supernumerary nipples may occur. They appear as slightly pigmented linear dimples with palpable breast nodules (Kenner & Lott, 2007). The amount of breast tissue relates to gestational age. The internipple distance is approximately 25 percent of the chest circumference in the term infant (Kenner & Lott, 2007). Widely spaced nipples are associated with a variety of congenital syndromes, including multiple congenital anomalies/mental retardation syndrome, Leopard syndrome, Noonan's syndrome, Down syndrome (trisomy 21) and Kleinfellter Syndrome. The term infant has a stippled areola with a raised edge. Breast tissue is palpable on both sides. Sometimes a white, milky discharge occurs toward the end of the first week of life. Hypertrophy of the breast also may occur. These findings are acceptable and will resolve.

The nurse observes the chest for symmetry and expansion. Asymmetry is abnormal and may indicate a problem, such as diaphragmatic hernia or pneumothorax. The infant uses the diaphragm muscles for breathing and adapts to using the intercostal muscles with maturity. Use of abdominal muscles indicates respiratory distress. The expected respiratory rate is 40 to 60 breaths per minute for a full minute. The infant's state of consciousness influences respiratory rate. Deep sleep is associated with a fairly regular breathing pattern, and the awake state is characterized by irregular breathing. Because of the decreased compliance of the ribs, occasional mild subcostal retractions may occur in healthy neonates.

The nurse assesses the infant chest by inspection and palpation. The precordium is the area of the anterior chest under which the heart lies. The precordium is usually quiet. A bounding precordium usually is characteristic of a ventricular septal defect or a heart defect, such as patent ductus arteriosus (PDA) (Lott, 2007; Tappero & Honeyfield, 2003). The normal point of maximal impulse is on the left side in the fourth intercostal space, either at or to the left of the midclavicular line (Tappero & Honeyfield, 2003).

The heart is assessed for rate, rhythm, murmurs and character of sounds. The nurse auscultates and counts heart rate for 1 full minute. Brief episodes of cardiac deceleration followed by increased heart rate are common and acceptable. The average heart rate ranges from 120 to 160 beats per minute (Kenner & Lott, 2007).

Because of the rapid rate, it is difficult to evaluate newborn heart sounds. The first heart sound, best heard at the apex of the heart, is loud at birth and decreases during the first 48 hours of life. The second heart sound is loud and single at birth. About half of infants reveal splitting of the second heart sound after about 4 hours. Third and fourth heart sounds are rarely heard in the newborn period (Tappero & Honeyfield, 2003). Cardiac murmurs usually are heard shortly after birth. They typically are systolic murmurs of grade 1 or 2 out of 6 and are not associated with distress. The nurse describes a murmur by intensity, quality, shape, location and radiation. Murmurs commonly are heard before the ductus arteriosus closes completely. If a murmur persists for longer than 48 to 72 hours, it requires further evaluation (Kenner & Lott, 2007; Lott, 2007).

The nurse assesses the pulses when the infant is in a quiet state. Femoral pulses present bilaterally. The nurse compares femoral pulses with pulses in the upper extremities. Absence or decreased intensity of pulses indicates inadequate aortic blood flow, as seen with coarctation of the aorta, aortic stenosis and hypoplastic left-heart syndrome. Bounding pulses in any extremity require follow-up. They are usually present with PDA or other aortic runoff lesions (Lott, 2007; Tappero & Honeyfield, 2003).

Perfusion may be assessed by capillary refill. The nurse presses the skin over the abdomen or an extremity until the skin blanches. The number of seconds that elapse until the color returns to the area is the capillary refill time. Refill time should be <3 seconds (Kenner & Lott, 2007).

Abdomen

The nurse assesses the abdomen for contour, size, symmetry and umbilical cord location. The healthy infant's abdomen is soft, symmetrical and slightly rounded and moves in conjunction with the chest during respiration.

The umbilical cord of a healthy infant is shiny, pearly white and gelatinous. It contains Wharton's jelly, which protects the vessels. The cord also indicates nutritional status. LGA infants usually have a thick cord; SGA and postmature infants or infants with placental insufficiency usually have a small, thin cord. The nurse assesses the cord for two arteries and one vein. Absence of a vessel may indicate renal or cardiovascular anomalies. The stump should not ooze or bleed. The stump darkens and shrivels as it dries, usually falling off within 10 days to 14 days (Tappero & Honeyfield, 2003).

The nurse palpates the abdomen to locate vital organs and any masses. When the infant's abdomen is assessed, the nurse flexes the knees and legs toward the hips to allow relaxation of the abdominal muscles (Erdman & Erdman, 2007). The infant should urinate by 24 hours of age and have a bowel movement by 48 hours.

The nurse teaches parents about the color and consistency of meconium stools and the amount of urine expected. Parents should understand how stool and urine changes reflect the infant's feeding pattern.

Liver

The liver is palpated 1 cm to 2 cm inferior to the right costal margin at the midclavicular line. Palpation begins just above the iliac crest on the right by placing the palm surface of the fingers parallel to the costal margin. The nurse then gently palpates in a progressively caudal fashion. This technique allows the nurse to then palpate the left side of the abdomen for the spleen (Tappero & Honeyfield, 2003). The liver edge should be firm and sharp. A large, soft liver with poorly defined edges may indicate congestive heart failure. Respiratory disease with hyperexpansion may cause lower-than-normal liver edge. A liver located >3 cm below the right costal margin may indicate right-sided heart failure in a term infant (Tappero & Honeyfield, 2003).

Spleen

In infants, only the tip of the spleen can be felt; in many cases the spleen is not palpable. A palpable spleen more than 1 cm below the left costal margin is abnormal (Brown, 2007).

Kidneys

The nurse examines the kidneys for shape, texture and size (Altimier, Quatman & Howard, 2007). Neonatal kidneys may be difficult to find (Kenner & Lott, 2007). To palpate the left kidney, the nurse places the right hand beneath the left lumbar region and explores the left flank with the thumb or fingers of the left hand. The procedure is reversed to palpate the right kidney. Kidneys are smooth and firm to touch when palpated. The length of the kidney in the term infant is 4.5 cm to 5.0 cm from the upper to the lower pole.

Anogenital Area

The anus is evaluated for patency and tone. Gentle stroking of the anal area produces constriction of the sphincter, known as the anal wink.

Male Genitalia

The nurse checks the glans, urethral opening, prepuce and shaft of the penis. The penis in the term male infant is approximately 3.5 cm from the pubic bone to the tip of the glans, excluding the foreskin (Tappero & Honeyfield, 2003). The nurse retracts the foreskin to inspect the urethral opening. The opening should be large enough to allow urination. The urine stream should be forceful and straight (Kenner & Lott, 2007).

The nurse examines the infant for hypospadias, where the urethral opening is on the ventral penile surface. Hypospadias results from incomplete development of the anterior urethra (Tappero & Honeyfield, 2003). It is a contraindication for circumcision (Altimier, Quatman & Howard, 2007). Hypospadias is common, occurring in approximately 8.2 infants per 1,000 births (Altimier, Quatman & Howard, 2007).

The nurse examines the scrotum for size, rugation and the presence of testes. The male infant has a fully rugated scrotum with brownish pigmentation. On palpation, testes are firm, smooth and comparatively equal in size. The testes begin descent at about 27 weeks gestation; they should be descended by 34 weeks to 39 weeks (Kenner & Lott, 2007).

Female Genitalia

The nurse examines the labia, clitoris, urethral opening and external vaginal vault. In the term female infant, the labia majora completely covers the labia minora. It is acceptable to see a mucoid discharge, which is sometimes accompanied by a small amount of blood. The discharge is caused by withdrawal of maternal estrogen after delivery (Tappero & Honeyfield, 2003). The clitoris is located superior to the vaginal opening and appears relatively large. Hymenal tags may be seen. Tags usually disappear several weeks after birth (Altimier, Quatman & Howard, 2007).

Skeletal System

Spine
The nurse observes and palpates the curvature of the spine and performs passive flexion, extension and lateral bending. The back should be symmetrical on both sides and between the two scapulae. The healthy spine is flexible and straight. Defects, such as pits, hair tufts, dimples or meningomyelocele, should not be present. The vertebrae should be palpable without discomfort.

Extremities
Extremities are assessed for symmetry, degree of flexion and presence of defects and fractures. The extremities should have full range of motion and move symmetrically.

Upper Extremities

The nurse inspects and palpates the clavicles for size, contour, masses and crepitance. Signs of fractured clavicles include crepitance and decreased shoulder movement. The nurse examines the scapulae for contour, symmetry and shoulder movement and the humeri for length and contour. The elbow, forearm and wrist are assessed for number, size and bone contour. The nurse carefully evaluates the hands for shape, size and posture and fingers for number, shape and length. Healthy fingers are equally spaced and without webbing. Palmar creases may indicate certain conditions, such as Down syndrome or Trisomy 21.

Lower Extremities

The nurse assesses a newborn's posture with hip and knee flexion. The hips are put through full range of motion to rule out congenital hip dysplasia. Asymmetry of skin folds in the gluteal and femoral regions suggests dislocation (Tappero & Honeyfield, 2003). The nurse performs the Ortolani maneuver and Barlow's test to check for congenital hip dysplasia. The Ortolani maneuver reduces a dislocated femoral head into the acetabulum, and the Barlow maneuver reflects the ability of the femoral head to be dislocated. Asymmetrical creases in the buttocks suggest congenital hip dysplasia.

The knees are examined for contour, range of motion and presence of the patella. The lower legs are examined for length and shape. The nurse inspects the feet for number and spacing of toes and the soles for creasing.

Sleep and Activity Patterns

A term, nonstressed neonate follows a predictable pattern of behavior during the initial hours after birth. The first 6 hours to 8 hours after birth are called the transitional period. During this time, the newborn exhibits behavioral changes related to sleep/ awake states and response to stimuli. The newborn also experiences physiologic variations during three phases: (1) reactivity immediately after birth, (2) relative inactivity and (3) a second episode of reactivity. The sequence is consistent among newborns, but the timing and length of each varies and is influenced by factors including maternal medications, length of labor and the extrauterine environment.

During the initial period of reactivity (the first hour after birth), the newborn is alert and active. The infant exhibits a strong desire to suck, providing an excellent opportunity to initiate breastfeeding. It is a good time for parent-newborn interaction and bonding. Delaying prophylactic eye medication until after this period allows the newborn to visually respond to parents. The neonate may be tachypneic (up to 80 breaths per minute) and tachycardic (up to 180 beats per minute) and may exhibit mild to moderate chest-wall retractions, grunting and flaring. Acrocyanosis is expected during this time, but central cyanosis is not. Other signs of risk include apnea >15 seconds, asymmetrical chest-wall movement, unequal breath sounds, lethargy and excessive salivation and mucous. These risks need further evaluation and may require immediate intervention and treatment.

Responsiveness to surroundings gradually decreases until the neonate falls asleep, usually 2 to 3 hours after birth. This period of relative inactivity may last from just a few minutes to several hours. The newborn shows little interest in external stimuli and arouses with difficulty. Respiratory rate may increase during sleep, with the heart rate ranging from 120 to140 beats per minute.

The second episode of reactivity begins when the newborn awakens from this first sleep. It lasts from 4 hours to 6 hours. The infant is alert and responsive again, and heart and respiratory rates increase. The first urine and meconium stool often are passed during this period. Heart and respiratory rates stabilize and become more regular.

Infant State Assessment

Assessment of infant state is an appropriate and important aspect of neonatal care (Louw & Maree, 2005). Evaluation of newborn behavior incorporates assessment of state, reactions to stimulation and the newborn's ability to move from one state to another. The state organization system incorporates different ranges of sleep-awake states. Brazelton's (1984) neonatal behavioral assessment scale (NBAS) is a scoring system that assesses two sleep states and four awake states: deep sleep, light sleep, drowsy, quiet alert, active alert and crying.

State of consciousness affects newborn behavior and physiological parameters. A state-organized infant can transition between states and has the physiological and behavioral ability to reach or withdraw from any state. Organized state behavior indicates general well-being and CNS integrity. It also is a measure of the newborn's response to external stimuli.

The quiet alert state is the optimal state for feeding and for parent-infant interaction (Holditch-Davis, Blackburn & VandenBerg, 2003). It also is the best state for a gestational age exam.

The March of Dimes has two online, interactive modules on infant states and behavior. *Understanding the Behavior of Term Infants* (Blackburn & Bakewell-Sachs, 2004) offers continuing education for registered nurses. It includes information on states of the term newborn and infant temperament, behavior, reflexes and cues; state modulation and self-regulation; changes in sleep and wake patterns during early infancy; and nursing interventions for new parents. For a free preview, nurses can visit marchofdimes.com/nursing.

The second module, *Understanding Your Newborn* (Blackburn & Bakewell-Sachs, 2007), is designed for parents. It explains how infants communicate and respond to the world around them. Topics include how babies signal that they're hungry, tired, don't feel well or want to play; how sleep patterns change over time; how a newborn responds and moves; and how to manage a crying baby. To access this free module, parents can visit marchofdimes.com/newborn.

Newborn Screening and Genetic Testing

Newborn and metabolic screening programs and newborn genetic testing first became feasible in 1962 when Dr. Robert Guthrie (Guthrie & Susi, 1963) developed a simple, cost-effective screening method using a small amount of blood collected on filter paper. Today, screening programs are mandatory in most states and are used to identify infants who are at risk for phenylketonuria (PKU), congenital hypothyroidism (CH), other metabolism errors and hemoglobinopathies. Newborn screening allows providers to detect and treat conditions early. If undetected and untreated, some conditions may cause developmental delays, mental retardation, learning disabilities and organ damage.

> **Evaluation of newborn behavior incorporates assessment of state, reactions to stimulation and the newborn's ability to move from one state to another.**

Some states require 30 or more tests because they are easy to administer and analyze through tandem mass spectrometry or ms/ms (two mass spectrometers connected by a common chamber that breaks a molecule into pieces). The National Newborn Screening and Genetics Resource Center (1997) (genes-r-us.uthscsa.edu) offers a listing by state of required newborn screening tests. The March of Dimes (2006) recommends newborn screening for 29 conditions (Table 14).

The March of Dimes recommends newborn screening for 29 conditions.

Table 14. March of Dimes Newborn Screening Recommendations	
Type	**Disorder**
Organic acid metabolism disorders	• Isovaleric acidemia (IVA) • Glutaric acidemia (GA I) • 3-OH 3-CH3 glutaric aciduria (HMG) • Multiple carboxylase deficiency (MCD) • Methylmalonic acidemia due to mutase deficiency (MUT) • Methylmalonic acidemia (Cbl A,B) • 3-methylcrotonyl-CoA carboxylase deficiency (3MCC) • Propionic acidemia PROP • Beta-ketothiolase deficiency (BKT)
Fatty acid oxidation disorders	• Medium-chain acyl-CoA dehydrogenase deficiency (MCAD) • Very long-chain acyl-CoA dehydrogenase deficiency (VLCAD) • Long-chain L-3-OH acyl-CoA dehydrogenase deficiency (LCHAD) • Trifunctional protein deficiency (TFP) • Carnitine uptake defect (CUD)
Amino acid metabolism disorders	• Phenylketonuria (PKU) • Maple syrup urine disease (MSUD) • Homocystinuria due to CBS deficiency (HCY) • Citrullinemia (CIT) • Argininosuccinic academia (ASA) • Tyrosinemia type I (TYR I)
Hemoglobinopathies	• Sickle cell anemia (Hb SS) • Hemoglobin S/beta-thalassemia (Hb S/Th) • Hemoglobin S/C disease [DEFINE] (Hb S/C)
Other	• Congenital hypothyroidism (CH) • Biotinidase deficiency (BIOT) • Congenital adrenal hyperplasia due to 21-hydroxylase deficiency (CAH) • Classical galactosemia (GALT) • Hearing loss (HEAR) • Cystic fibrosis (CF)

March of Dimes, 2006

Many conditions for which tests are possible are not treatable, nor can their course be altered. However, when the course can be altered or the condition successfully treated, screening is an essential part of newborn care (Kenner, Gallo & Bryant, 2005; Kenner & Moran, 2005).

Policies regarding parental informed consent for newborn screening differ. Twenty-eight states require informed consent; the remaining 22 states consider newborn screening to be covered by the consent-to-treat document that parents or guardians sign when an infant is born or as part of the maternal consent upon admission to the maternal-child unit (Kenner & Moran, 2005). AWHONN (2004) recommends parental consent even when the tests are mandatory. As health care shifts to a patient/family-centered focus, parents may want the ability to make their own decisions about newborn screening, especially for tests that identify conditions that are untreatable or unalterable.

Sample collection for screening occurs between 48 hours and 72 hours after birth. This window allows time for metabolic changes to occur and for the newborn to ingest formula or breastmilk (protein) so that PKU screening is accurate. It is also early enough to identify conditions, such as galactosemia and maple syrup urine disease, before the onset of life-threatening symptoms. However, with early discharge at 12 hours to 24 hours, providers may need to conduct the test and repeat it later, if necessary. Some states require that an initial sample be obtained immediately before discharge, with a second sample at 7 days to 14 days of life. Birth centers and home-birth attendants should follow screening procedures mandated by their state.

Perinatal and neonatal nurses should know the screenings required by their state, including signs, symptoms and outcomes of untreated conditions; criteria for repeat tests; available treatments; and hereditary patterns (Kenner & Moran, 2005).

Family History Tool

The Human Genome Project has reframed the concept of health. Using the genetic lens to examine risk factors, the nurse and other health care providers can make recommendations for health promotion. One way to identify genetic risk factors for an infant is to do a thorough assessment, including a 3-generation family history. The Centers for Disease Control and Prevention (CDC) National Office of Public Health Genomics (2006a) advocates the family history as an important tool for preventative medicine. Families are encouraged to complete their own family history and keep it as part of their health records. An interactive family history form can be found at https://familyhistory.hhs.gov/selfInfo.cfm.

Thermoregulation in the Newborn

Thermoregulation is the balance between heat production and heat loss; the goal is to maintain thermal equilibrium. Thermoregulation is vital to the newborn and is entirely managed by nurses. Nurses must understand mechanisms of heat loss and gain, be knowledgeable about assessment and intervention, and correctly interpret body temperature.

Neonatal thermoregulation is closely linked to the infant's survival and health status (Kenner & Lott, 2007). Table 15 provides an overview of infants at risk for problems with thermoregulation. Understanding the concept of heat exchange and the physiology of human thermoregulation is crucial to providing a thermoneutral environment for the infant. The human body increases or decreases heat production to maintain core body temperature. The newborn's response range to environmental temperature is narrower than an adult's, and neonatal skin receptors are more sensitive than those of an adult. Neonatal skin receptors are located throughout the body but concentrated in the trigeminal area of the face. The newborn has two types of peripheral receptors—one for detecting cool temperatures and one for detecting warm temperatures. The skin contains 10 times more cool receptors than warm ones; therefore, the cool receptors are more

Table 15. Term Infants at Risk for Problems in Thermoregulation	
Infant Category	**Basis for Risk**
Infants with neurologic problems	Alteration in hypothalamic control
Infants with endocrine problems	• Impaired brown adipose tissue (BAT) metabolism due to inadequate catecholamine and/or hormones • Decreased substrate for energy
Hypoglycemic infants	• Decreased metabolic response to cold stress • Inability to increase oxygen consumption or minute ventilation further
Infants with cardiorespiratory problems	• Inability to increase metabolic rate and reduce metabolic response to cold • Impaired BAT metabolism due to hypoxemia • Inadequate caloric intake to meet metabolic demands • Increased risk of metabolic acidosis • Increased temperature loss through evaporation from the lungs
Infants with congenital anomalies, such as meningomyelocele, omphalocele and gastroschisis	• Increased surface area for heat loss • Increased evaporative losses
SGA infants	• Decreased subcutaneous fat insulation • Increased surface area for body weight
Sedated infants or maternal intrapartal analgesia	• Higher basal metabolic rate and energy demands • Limited physical activity to generate heat • Maternal diazepam or meperidine associated with decreased newborn temperature

Blackburn, 2003. Reprinted with permission.

important in initiating responses to temperatures. Heat production in the neonate is related more to a decrease in skin temperature than core temperature; in the adult, it is related to a decrease in core temperature (Uebel, 2007).

The fetus moves from a warm, wet intrauterine environment to a cool, dry extrauterine environment. The newborn experiences rapid heat loss after birth, primarily through evaporation, with a fall in temperature of 2 C to 3 C (Blackburn, 2007). Cold stress occurs when heat loss overwhelms the newborn's ability to produce heat. Poor thermal stability in the neonate primarily is caused by excessive heat loss, rather than by impaired heat production.

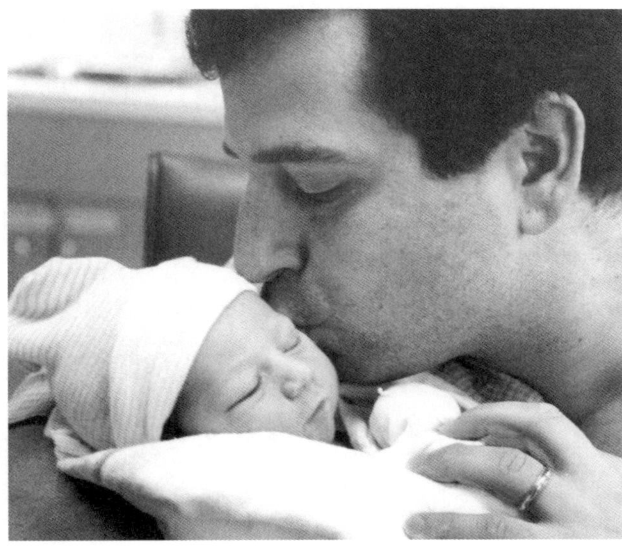

Newborns are most likely to become cold stressed in the first 4 hours after birth. When neonatal skin receptors sense a cooler environmental temperature, norepinephrine is released through the posterior hypothalamus by sympathetic nervous control. This release causes blood vessels in the skin to constrict, decreasing blood flow to the skin and keeping heat in the body. Because the facial area has many skin receptors, blowing cool air across the face may initiate this response.

Family-centered care is valuable in maintaining thermoregulation in infants. The infant may better tolerate being swaddled or having kangaroo care than being in an isolette or radiant warmer. Swaddling and kangaroo care create a smaller difference in air temperature than does an isolette or radiant warmer. Holding their baby for extended periods of time gives moms and dads self-confidence as parents and helps them feel in control of infant care.

Heat Loss Mechanisms

The human body transfers heat within itself and externally to and from the environment. The four avenues of heat exchange can be summarized by the four traditional elements of earth, air, fire and water (Chandra & Baumgart, 2005a). Conduction (earth) is the transfer of heat when two solid objects are in surface-to-surface contact. Convection (air) is the transfer of heat between areas that are in contact with each other but that are not solid. Radiation (fire) is the transfer of heat from a warmer object to a cooler object but without contact. Evaporation (water) is heat loss caused by evaporation of water from the skin. These four mechanisms account for all avenues of heat loss from the body (Table 16). All methods except evaporation assist in heat gain. All four methods are critical when considering a thermal-neutral environment (Uebel, 2007).

Table 16. Sources of Heat Loss and Overheating and Nursing Interventions		
Mechanisms	**Sources of Heat Loss/Overheating**	**Interventions**
Evaporation	Wet body surface and hair at delivery and with bathing	• Thoroughly dry infant, especially the head, immediately after birth with a warm blanket. • Use insulated caps or hooded blankets. • Replace wet blankets with warm, dry ones. • Place dried infant skin-to-skin on mother's chest and cover with warmed blanket. • Delay initial bath until body temperature has stabilized. • Bathe in warm, draft-free environment and dry immediately; bathe under a radiant warmer.
Conduction	Cool mattress, blanket, scale, table, equipment or clothing	• Place warm blankets on scales, X-ray plates, other surfaces in direct contact with infant. • Preheat blankets, clothing, radiant warmer and equipment before use. • Heating pads, hot water bottles, chemical bags. • Transport infants in prewarmed incubators. • Avoid placing infant on any surface that is warmer than the infant.
Convection	Cool air temperature in room, hallways or outside air	• Maintain room temperature at levels adequate to provide a safe thermal environment for infant (72 to 76 degrees F). • Swaddle with warm blankets (except when under radiant warmer), use insulated caps or hooded blankets.
	Convective air-flow incubator	Monitor incubator air temperature to avoid temperatures warmer than the infant's body temperature.
	Drafts from air vents, windows, doors, heaters, fans, air conditions	• Place infants away from air vents, drafts and other sources of moving air currents. • Use side guards on radiant warmers to decrease crosscurrent air flow across infant.
	Cold oxygen flow (especially near facial thermal receptors)	Use warm and humidified oxygen; minimize use of cool, dry free-flow oxygen.
	Placement near cold or hot external windows or walls, placement in direct sunlight	• Place incubators, cribs and radiant warmers away from external walls and windows, and direct sunlight. • Use thermal shades on external windows.
Radiation	Cold incubator walls	Prewarm incubators, radiant warmers, heat shields.
	Heat lamps	Avoid use whenever possible; if used, monitor temperature every 10 to 15 minutes to avoid burns.

Blackburn, 2003. Reprinted with permission.

Infant heat is transferred to the air, and the warmed air rises. The amount of skin exposed to the environment affects how much heat is lost. Therefore, overheated infants assume an extended position, and cold-stressed infants assume a flexed position.

Heat Dissipation

Infants have a limited ability to compensate for heat stress. The body responds to overheating by vasodilatation in the skin, which increases heat loss from the blood. Vasodilatation occurs when the anterior hypothalamus senses an increase in central or peripheral temperature. The anterior hypothalamus inhibits the posterior hypothalamus from sending sympathetic impulses that cause vasoconstriction.

At certain core body temperatures, the anterior hypothalamus signals the release of acetylcholine in the sweat glands to produce sweat. Sweating causes evaporative heat loss. An adult can remove 10 times the basal rate of heat production via sweat. When exposed to excessive temperatures, the neonate may vasodilate but has limited ability to sweat. Infant sweat glands are capable of about one-third of the response of adult sweat glands. The infant may not always appear to be sweating, but evaporative heat loss may increase. Sweat glands in the forehead are the most mature and may be the only visible signs of sweat in a newborn.

The largest amount of heat loss in the first week of life is caused by evaporation due to immaturity of the skin. After birth the skin matures quickly. Heat dissipation also can occur when the body position changes, increasing the amount of skin exposed to the environment. The overheated adult or infant assumes a flaccid, extended position to increase heat transfer from the skin to the environment. The risk of neonatal hyperthermia is high in warm, humid environments. Unlike in adults, when the infant's capability to transfer heat to the environment is exceeded, the metabolic rate increases, resulting in excess heat production. This can lead to a fatal hyperthermia.

Providers frequently use head coverings to minimize newborn heat loss. The newborn's head represents 21 percent of the total body surface area and accounts for a significant proportion of total heat loss (Blackburn, 2007). In addition, brain heat production accounts for 55 percent of the total metabolic heat production. The most effective head coverings include: wool with a gauze and cotton lining; Thinsulate® (polyolefin microfibers commonly used to manufacture winter outerwear); and cotton/polyester fill or terry cloth. Head coverings are most effective in a cool environment and less effective in a thermoneutral environment or with use of infant servo control. Servo control entails use of a temperature probe on the infant's skin that automatically regulates the bed temperature in accordance with preset temperature limits. Head coverings and clothing interfere with radiant heat loss and gain and are not appropriate for infants under radiant warmers (Blackburn, 2007).

Heat Production

The human body responds to cold in three ways: (1) voluntary muscular activity, (2) shivering and (3) chemical or nonshivering thermogenesis.

Vasoconstriction is one aspect of voluntary muscle control to overcome hypothermia. Another is the ability to produce movement. Movement increases metabolism, which increases heat production. The body can assume a flexed position to decrease the amount of skin exposed to the cooler environment, effectively conserving heat for the body. These mechanisms are functional in the healthy neonate.

Shivering is the chief method of heat production in the adult; however, it is inefficient in the term newborn.

Chemical or nonshivering thermogenesis is important in the neonate but is almost absent in the adult. It depends on a type of fat called brown fat that develops in the fetus at 26 to 30 weeks gestation and continues until birth. It is located around the scapulae, across the clavicle line, along the spinal cord, in the axilla, around the thymus, around the great vessels and in the padding of the kidney. Heat generation is essentially the metabolism of brown fat. The infant can increase metabolic rate and heat production with brown fat metabolism, but the process is limited. Prolonged cold stress can delete brown fat.

A term infant can use increased movement, vasoconstriction and brown-fat metabolism for several hours after birth without intervention. After this time, brown fat and glycogen stores are depleted due to a lack of glucose immediately after birth. Glucose is paramount for metabolism of brown fat. Hypoglycemia inhibits an infant's ability to increase heat production. Also, the infant stressed in utero may have depleted his glycogen and brown-fat stores. Another limiting factor may be oxygen, especially if the neonate has respiratory compromise. Fat metabolism requires oxygen, and brown fat consumes more oxygen than the heart muscle does. The more heat the infant requires, the more oxygen he needs. As the compromised infant develops hypoxia, anaerobic metabolism occurs with the build-up of lactic acid and acidosis. Acidosis and hypoxemia contribute to pulmonary hypertension.

Illness and other conditions affect the infant's ability to produce or conserve heat. To produce heat, the infant requires intact central and peripheral nervous systems, the ability to move around, and sufficient glucose and oxygen. Many circumstances impair these factors. For example, developmental status may limit the infant's ability to move. Sedated or paralyzed infants have limited movement to increase heat production. A decrease in CNS functioning, as seen in asphyxia or intraventricular hemorrhage, may change the ability of the hypothalamus to respond to changes in environmental temperature. If the mother receives analgesia during labor, the infant's metabolism is slowed for the first few days of life, making it difficult to produce energy for heat production.

Temperature

At birth, the neonate's temperature is slightly higher (about 0.5 C) than the maternal core body temperature. If the mother has a fever, the infant's temperature may be slightly increased. At birth, the neonate's temperature may decrease at a rate of 0.2 C to 1.0 C per minute, mainly through convective and evaporative heat loss. AAP and ACOG (2007) have established the following norms: a rectal or auxiliary temperature of 36.5 C to 37.5 C and a skin temperature of 36 C to 36.5 C. However, it is not uncommon to record a body temperature as low as 35.5 C at or immediately after birth. The infant's body temperature should be stable with a change 0.2 C to 0.3 C per hour. The temperature may fluctuate as 0.5 C in a day.

The anterior hypothalamus, the central thermostat for the body, works to maintain core body temperature within a 0.6 C range. It does this through heat- and cool-sensitive neurons triggered by change in core body temperature. Signals from the anterior hypothalamus, the skin and deep organ receptors influence the posterior hypothalamus to control heat-producing, heat-conserving and heat-dissipating activities of the body.

Thermoneutral Environment

To avoid physiologic consequences of cold stress and hyperthermia, providers must keep the infant in a thermoneutral environment. A thermoneutral environment is a range of environmental temperatures in which an infant's metabolic rate is at a minimum and body temperature is maintained (Chandra & Baumgart, 2005b). Above this range, the infant is unable to dissipate heat and water loss and metabolic rate increases. The body can reach extremely high temperatures, causing seizures and death. Below the range, the infant must increases his metabolic rate to produce more heat. This can deplete oxygen and glucose. If an infant reaches a metabolic rate that he cannot surpass, the body begins to cool. Without intervention, death from hypothermia may result.

Room temperature usually is around 25 C; while comfortable for the mother, this temperature provides an environment for convective, and probably radiant, heat loss for the infant. At birth in a 25 C room, the infant requires 200 Kcal/kg/min to match the heat loss (Knobel, Wimmer & Holbert, 2005). Placing the infant under a prewarmed radiant warmer, wrapping in warm, dry blankets, and placing a hat on the head helps decrease heat loss. A healthy, term, AGA infant, when clothed and fed, can regulate body temperature in cooler environments without compensating growth for 2 to 3 days. Room temperature for cesarean birth is usually colder than in a regular labor and delivery room. Measures to prevent infant heat loss are key in the immediate care of a newborn after cesarean birth (Uebel, 20007).

Radiant Warmer

Radiant warmers use radiant heat to warm an infant. Radiant heat gained by an infant can offset convective, conductive and evaporative heat loss. Radiant warmers allow easy access to and visibility of the infant and are less of a barrier to parental bonding than incubators.

The risk of infant hyperthermia can be high under a radiant warmer, especially when providers ignore or silence alarms or place the warmer on manual mode instead of servo mode (infant servo control). According to Flenady and Woodgate (2003), there is no evidence to support increased oxygen consumption when a radiant warmer is used for newborn thermoregulation. When the probe is placed over bony prominences, extremities or excoriated areas, readings vary from the infant's actual temperature. Probe placement is best on the upper right quadrant of the abdomen or between the umbilicus and pubis, provided the infant is supine

(Blackburn, 2007). A reflective patch must be used over the skin probe; otherwise, the probe may sense a higher temperature than the skin because of infrared heat sources, such as phototherapy, heaters or lights.

Temperature Assessment

Rectal temperature has long been the standard for core temperature measurement. However, this method carries a high risk of rectal perforation. The depth of the thermometer in the rectum can affect the temperature reading. A depth of 3 cm avoids rectal perforation; however, 4 cm to 5 cm is needed for accurate temperature measurement.

For neonates and infants, axillary temperatures closely correlate with rectal temperatures and are safer for the infant. Therefore, axillary temperatures should be used unless otherwise indicated. Axillary temperature, on average, is 0.4 C less than rectal temperature (Kenner, 2003). Axillary temperature may be higher because the axilla has brown fat stores that produce heat that radiates to the skin. For the axillary temperature to be accurate, nurses must hold the thermometer firmly against the skin.

Hyperthermia

Infant hyperthermia is caused by an overheated environment or fever. Nurses must recognize the difference between the two causes to avoid the risk, discomfort and cost of a septic workup. Accurate documentation of skin, core and air temperatures can aid in the diagnosis.

Bacterial pyrogens or endotoxins can raise the hypothalamic set point of the body. The body responds by trying to conserve and produce heat to increase the core temperature to the new set point. The blood vessels constrict to keep heat in the body core. Shivers and chills associated with fever are the mature body's attempt to increase metabolism to warm the body. The body assumes a hypermetabolic state, using oxygen and glucose to produce heat.

Because infants are unable to shiver, metabolism of brown fat may increase to raise body temperature. Also, the infant's response to the increased set point may be immature; thus, temperature may lower in response to bacterial toxins. In overwhelming sepsis, bacterial endotoxins may lead to vasodilatation, causing the infant to lose more heat and become hypothermic. A difference >3.5 C between infant core and skin temperatures, even when the infant is normothermic, may be a sign of overwhelming sepsis.

An infant with hyperthermia related to sepsis presents differently than an infant with hyperthermia caused by a hot environment. In febrile infants, core temperature increases before skin temperature. Because of vasoconstriction to conserve heat, the infant has cool extremities, which may appear dusky, mottled or pale. The rectal temperature is warmer than the skin temperature by >3.5 C, and the abdominal skin temperature is >3 C warmer than the skin temperature of the foot (Kenner, 2003). After making sure the skin-temperature reading is correct, the nurse may need to increase the air temperature to increase Term skin temperature. Because the infant is hypermetabolic, nurses also must assess other indicators, including increased oxygen requirement and presence of hypoglycemia, metabolic acidosis or lethargy.

When an infant is hyperthermic from an overheated environment, skin temperature increases first, followed by core temperature. The increases are related to the skin-air temperature gradient—when the air temperature is greater than the skin temperature, the infant gains convective heat. The infant placed next to a hot, solid object also may gain radiant heat. The infant's body tries to lose heat by vasodilatation and becomes flushed with warm extremities. To prevent a rise in core temperature, the infant must be cooled. The infant is at risk for dehydration, acidosis, seizures and death.

Hypothermia

Infants differ in their responses to cool body temperature. Some infants with a body temperature of 35.5 C may be sleeping and content; others may show signs of cold stress. This difference may be attributed to the hypothalamic set point of each infant. The infant's body must recognize lower body temperature as a stress and respond by increasing metabolism to increase heat production. One of the earliest signs of heat conservation is vasoconstriction. The infant is pale and mottled with cool extremities and feeds poorly.

The cold-stressed infant may have an acceptable body temperature but may be hypermetabolic to maintain that temperature. Because the bedside nurse cannot measure metabolic rate, it is difficult to measure the energy necessary to maintain a core body temperature. A quick way to estimate whether the cold-stressed infant is in a neutral thermal environment is to ensure that the environmental temperature is not <2.5 C cooler than the infant's skin temperature. Nurses must remember that environmental temperature does not equal air temperature because of radiant heat loss. Environmental temperature may be 1 C to 2 C cooler than air temperature. The difference in air and environmental temperatures can be accounted for by measuring the ambient air temperature surrounding the infant.

Rewarming the Cold-stressed Infant

Nurses must carefully rewarm a cold-compromised infant. Warming too quickly may precipitate apnea in the infant. When the skin temperature warms too quickly, vasodilatation occurs, which may cause pooling of the blood in the extremities, leading to a decrease in blood pressure. When an infant is rewarmed, nurses closely monitor core and skin temperatures; skin temperature should not be warmer than core temperature by more than 1 C. The nurse rewarms the infant by swaddling, initiating skin-to-skin contact between infant and parent or placing the infant in an incubator or radiant-heat warmer.

The nurse slows the rewarming process if the infant becomes apneic or if the blood pressure decreases. An infant in an environment with an air temperature of 38 C requires constant nursing care to prevent hyperthermia. When skin servo control is used, the nurse may lightly swaddle a cold infant to decrease heat loss as long as the blanket does not interfere with the skin probe. This infant also may benefit from wearing a hat.

Newborn Problems: Assessment and Management

Respiratory Distress

Respiratory distress is a common neonatal complication. It decreases oxygenation and carbon dioxide exchange, which affect all body organs and tissues if prolonged. Respiratory distress occurs when there is an obstruction or malformation or other medical or systemic problems. It can develop as a complication of transition to extrauterine life.

The term newborn with upper airway congestion and minor airway infections may experience tremendous resistance, placing the infant at risk for increased work of breathing, muscle fatigue and respiratory failure (Blackburn, 2007). Trauma or infection of the upper airway passages may cause edema, which can lead to obstruction and decreased airflow. Airway constriction in the term newborn causes nasal flaring, retractions and tachypnea (Blackburn, 2007). Chest-wall retractions (subcostal, intercostal suprasternal) and use of accessory muscles occur when there is increased work of breathing, indicating a primary pulmonary disorder. Unequal breath sounds, diminished air entry and adventitious sounds, such as crackles, wheezes and rhonchi, are further evidence of a pulmonary problem.

Care of a newborn with respiratory distress requires basic understanding of the causes of the disease processes. The three most common respiratory conditions that cause respiratory distress in the term newborn are pneumonia, transient tachypnea of the newborn (TTN) and meconium aspiration syndrome (MAS).

Pneumonia

Pneumonias may be of viral, bacterial or other infectious origin. Transmission can occur transplacentally or by ascending infection following rupture of the membranes. Organisms in neonatal pneumonia most commonly associated with maternal amnionitis include Group B streptococcus (GBS), Escherichia coli (E. coli) and Haemophilus influenzae (H. influenzae). Less commonly involved are Streptococcus viridans (S. viridans), Listeria monocytogenes (L. monocytogenes) and anaerobes. The resulting inflammatory process disrupts the barrier function of the pulmonary endothelium, leading to abnormal protein permeability and edema of lung tissue (Barnett & Klein, 2006). Tachypnea (prolonged grunting and retractions beyond the immediate transition period) and temperature instability warrant further evaluation.

TTN

TTN occurs in approximately 1 percent of all deliveries (Risken, Abend-Weinger, Risken-Mashiah, Kugelman & Bader, 2005). Avery and colleagues (1966) first described TTN as delayed lung fluid clearance, a significant cause of respiratory distress in the newborn period. Contributing factors include maternal oversedation and cesarean birth without a trial of labor. Delayed absorption of fetal lung fluid is the underlying etiology.

Initially, the newborn is asymptomatic; however, shortly after birth the newborn shows symptoms, such as expiratory grunting, flaring of the nares and mild cyanosis. TTN usually occurs by 6 hours of age, with a respiratory rate as high as

The three most common respiratory conditions that cause respiratory distress in the term newborn are pneumonia, TTN and MAS.

140 breaths per minute. The newborn with TTN usually recovers within 24 to 48 hours with no major sequelae. Management consists of ruling out other causes of RDS and maintaining adequate oxygenation.

MAS

MAS develops in approximately 5 percent to 12 percent of infants delivered through meconium-strained amniotic fluid (MSAF) (Morris, 2007a). Aspirated meconium below the vocal cords and into the trachea causes a partial or complete obstruction of terminal airways and air sacs. Meconium creates a ball-valve effect, in which air enters the lower airways on inspiration but is trapped on exhalation (Morris, 2007a). MSAF may be present when the fetus has experienced hypoxia in utero. Risk factors for MSAF include postmaturity, SGA and fetal distress due to maternal hypertension, anemia or chronic disease. MSAF occurs in 8 percent to 19 percent of all deliveries, is more likely to happen in term or post-term births and occurs in one-third to one-half of pregnancies lasting longer than 42 weeks gestation (Fuloria & Wiswell, 2005).

Neonatal Glycemic Control

Hypoglycemia

Glucose Physiology and Etiology

Glucose homeostasis in the newborn depends on initiation of several hormonal and metabolic changes. Catecholamine levels increase after birth in response to a drop in body temperature, causing an increase in glucagon levels. The hormones involved in glucose balance either lower or elevate blood glucose (Table 17). Glucagon promotes the conversion of glycogen to glucose when there is an immediate need for energy (Blackburn, 2007). Hypoglycemia is caused by an inadequate supply of glucose, alterations in endocrine regulation or increased glucose regulation.

Table 17. Glucose-balancing Hormones	
Glucose-lowering hormone	Insulin
Glucose-elevating hormones	• Glucagon • Epinephrine • Glucocorticoids • Growth-factor hormones

Hypoglycemia in infants of diabetic mothers (IDMs) is related to poor maternal glucose control. When maternal diabetes is appropriately managed, IDMs have a lower incidence of neonatal hypoglycemia. Nurses should meticulously monitor maternal glucose levels during pregnancy so that normoglycemia is maintained before delivery. The March of Dimes nursing module *Diabetes in Pregnancy,* 3rd Edition (Kendrick, 2004) provides a comprehensive discussion of managing diabetes in the pregnant woman.

The interruption of nutrient transport from mother to baby following cord clamping forces the newborn to mobilize fuels to meet the metabolic demands of vital organs. The newborn must adjust to the cessation of maternal glucose supply, while responding to an increased demand for energy created by changes in body temperature, the stress of labor and initiation of breathing (Stanley & Pallotto,

2005). Glucose, the primary fuel, is stored as glycogen in the liver. During fetal life, glucose is diverted into glycogen storage in preparation for birth. Neonatal hypoglycemia occurs when metabolic adaptation is unable to maintain glucose homeostasis.

Term infants are unable to tolerate low glucose levels. Sick infants (hypoxia, ischemia, sepsis) may have greater glucose needs and be more vulnerable to the effects of hypoglycemia than healthy infants.

Definitions of hypoglycemia vary. The term is difficult to define, in part, because there is no correlation between blood-glucose levels and CNS effects. One commonly used definition is a blood-glucose level of <35 mg/dL for the full-term infant (Kenner & Lott, 2007). However, hypoglycemia is not a single number; rather, it is a trend of falling blood-glucose values. A full-term, healthy neonate maintains plasma-glucose levels between 40 mg/dL and 80 mg/dL during the first 6 hours of life; after 24 hours, normal plasma-glucose levels range between 45 mg/dL and 90 mg/dL (Kenner & Lott, 2007). When feeding is delayed for 6 hours after delivery, a term newborn's plasma-glucose level can fall to about 30 mg/dL. If a feeding is delayed for 2 days, the infant's fasting system matures and the preprandial values are rarely <50 mg/dL. The fasting system protects the newborn system and attempts to keep glucose levels stable.

Newborn hypoglycemia is either transient or persistent. Transient hypoglycemia is most common. It usually occurs within the first 48 hours of life, but it may not present until 72 hours or later (Blackburn, 2007). With persistent hypoglycemia, the condition does not resolve within hours to days of diagnosis, even with treatment. It is caused by errors of metabolism, hyperinsulinism secondary to beta cell hyperplasia, and endocrine disorders. Neonates who develop hypoglycemia in the first 24 hours of life typically are IDMs, IUGR, SGA or LGA, or those who show signs of stress (asphyxia, sepsis, hypothermia, respiratory distress). Table 18 identifies etiologies and time course of neonatal hypoglycemia.

Newborn hypoglycemia can be asymptomatic or symptomatic. It can be life-threatening and may cause adverse neurologic sequelae, such as seizures and learning disabilities (Katz & Stanley, 2005). The risk of brain damage or developmental consequences may be related to the duration and severity of the hypoglycemia (Stanley & Pallotto, 2005). Therefore, early assessment of newborns and early initiation of preventive measures are important. It is up to each institution to establish its own guidelines for newborn hypoglycemia screening.

Signs and Symptoms

In the newborn period, signs of hypoglycemia may be absent or subtle, even when blood-glucose levels are extremely low. When the plasma-glucose level reaches a concentration of approximately 40 mg/dL, signs and symptoms become apparent (Table 19). If hypoglycemia remains untreated, manifestations of cerebral dysfunction, such as irritability, seizures and coma, develop, with resultant permanent CNS damage.

Management

Anticipation and prevention are the goals in managing hypoglycemia. Nurses should routinely assess infants at risk for clinical signs and monitor blood glucose. All newborns should be fed within the first 2 hours of life (breast or bottle), and

Table 18. Neonatal Hypoglycemia: Etiologies and Time Course

Mechanism	Clinical Setting	Expected Duration
Decreased substrate availability	IUGR	Transient
	Prematurity	Transient
	Glycogen-storage disease	Transient
	Inborn errors of metabolism	Prolonged
Endocrine disturbances	IDM	Transient
Hyperinsulinemia	Beckwith-Wiedemann syndrome	Prolonged
	Erythroblastosis fetalis	Transient
	Exchange transfusion	Transient
	Islet cell dysplasia	Prolonged
	Maternal B-sympathomimetics	Transient
	Improperly placed umbilical artery catheter	Transient
Other endocrine disorders	Hypopituitarism	Prolonged
	Hypothyroidism	Persistent
	Adrenal insufficiency	Persistent
Increased utilization	Birth asphyxia	Transient
	Hypothermia	Transient
Miscellaneous/Multiple factors	Sepsis	Transient
	Congenital heart disease	Transient
	Polycythemia	Transient
	CNS abnormalities	Prolonged

McGowan, 1998. Reprinted with permission.

Table 19. Signs and Symptoms of Neonatal Hypoglycemia

- Tremors
- Jitteriness
- Hypotonia
- Poor feeding
- Lethargy
- Irregular respiration
- Apnea
- Cyanosis
- Hypothermia
- Seizures

earlier feedings should be considered for at-risk newborns (Gamblian, Weiland & Park, 2003). To prevent an increase in metabolic demand due to hypothermia, an adequate thermal environment is critical.

A confirmed lab value indicative of hypoglycemia may be treated with a bolus of 2 mL/kg of D10W, followed immediately by an infusion of 6 mg/kg/min to 8 mg/kg/min, to maintain a blood glucose level above 40 mg/dL (Katy & Stanley, 2005). Frequent monitoring of glucose level (glucometer, lab analysis) and close observation of hydration are critical (Katz & Stanley, 2005). Once an adequate blood-glucose level is achieved and maintained, it is not necessary to measure blood-glucose concentration repeatedly unless there is a reduction in exogenous glucose supply.

Enteral feedings, either breastmilk or formula, are important in the management of neonatal hypoglycemia. Breastmilk and formula provide more energy per mL than 10 percent dextrose and supply important nonglucose fuels, which are necessary in the glucose-sparing role for neurologic function (Katz & Stanley, 2005). Because breastmilk is more ketogenic than formula, breastfeeding is encouraged. Enteral feedings should not be discontinued or reduced when intravenous fluids are given. By maximizing enteral feeding intake and gradually reducing intravenous infusion rates, most newborns achieve glucose homeostasis.

Hyperglycemia

Hyperglycemia in the newborn usually is defined as a blood glucose level >125 mg/dL (whole blood) or 145 mg/dL to 150 mg/dL (plasma). Hyperglycemia occurs less frequently than hypoglycemia, but it can significantly alter neurodevelopment. Hyperglycemia most often occurs in preterm newborns; however, it is seen in term neonates with sepsis, decreased insulin sensitivity or respiratory distress. Hyperglycemia is negatively correlated with birthweight and positively correlated with the rate of glucose infusion. It is typically asymptomatic and detected on routine laboratory screening. Hyperglycemia may cause osmotic changes and fluid shifts within the CNS, with a risk of intraventricular hemorrhage and glycosuria, in which fluids are drawn from the intracellular to the extracellular space resulting in dehydration (Blackburn, 2007). Frequent monitoring of blood-glucose levels and a urine assessment for osmotic diuresis are necessary for follow-up management.

Perinatal and Neonatal Infections

Perinatal infections contribute to neonatal infections and, thus, morbidity, mortality and increased length of hospital stay. The fetus and neonate are particularly susceptible to infection. Immune system development begins early in gestation; however, many immunologic responses are not functional or function inadequately in the early newborn period (Blackburn, 2007). Incomplete mucosal defenses may allow pathogens to more readily colonize the newborn. Even when infected, most newborns do not produce detectable type-specific antibodies. Newborns are unable to effectively localize infection because of their inability to produce adequate phagocytes and deliver them to the infection site. Because of transplacental transfer of immunoglobulins, primarily IgG, the term newborn has temporary passive immunity against infectious organisms to which the mother has created antibodies. Decreased levels of IgA reduce defense against gastrointestinal and respiratory infections, and decreased levels of IgM reduce the newborn's defense against viral and gram-negative bacteria (Blackburn, 2007). The newborn's increased susceptibility to infection and decreased ability to respond to it make risk assessment and early identification vital to reducing morbidity and mortality. Table 20 identifies risks of immunologic immaturity. Table 21 identifies predisposing risk factors for infection in the term newborn.

Table 20. Risks of Immunologic Immaturity
• Generalized sepsis in the presence of bacterial infection
• Respiratory and gastrointestinal infections
• E. coli sepsis, rubella, syphilis, toxoplasmosis, CMV and other viral infections
• Fungal infections

Table 21. Predisposing Risk Factors for Newborn Infection	
Maternal	• Malnutrition • Lack of prenatal care • Substance abuse • TORCH infections • Peripartum maternal fever • Clinical amnionitis • Urinary tract infection at time of delivery • Vaginal colonization with GBS • Perineal colonization with E. coli • Prolonged rupture of membranes (>24 hours) • Sexually transmitted infection (STI)
Neonatal	• Prematurity • Perinatal asphyxia • Male sex • Concurrent neonatal disease • IUGR • Galactosemia • Congenital asplenia

Kenner & Lott, 2007. Reprinted with permission.

Maternal infection can be passed to the fetus and newborn transplacentally in utero through direct contact with contaminated secretions in the birth canal at delivery; postbirth infection can occur via contaminated breastmilk (Kenner & Lott, 2007). Intrapartal transmission occurs through aspiration of infected amniotic fluid or when vaginal flora ascends to the unprotected fetus following rupture of membranes (Kenner & Lott, 2007). Newborns with viral infections acquired during fetal life may not demonstrate clinical disease at birth (Kenner & Lott, 2007).

Neonatal bacterial sepsis is classified according to timing of clinical presentation. Early-onset infection usually presents within 24 hours of birth, but it can present up to the end of the first week of life. It progresses rapidly and has a 10 percent to 25 percent risk of mortality, even with appropriate therapy (Kenner & Lott, 2007). Bacteria associated with early-onset sepsis are present in the maternal vaginal flora, including GBS, H. influenzae, L. monocytogenes, E. coli and Streptococcus pneumoniae (S. pneumoniae). Late-onset sepsis usually presents after 2 weeks of age but can occur any time after the first week of life. It progresses more slowly and has a lower mortality than early-onset infection, but higher morbidity (Kenner & Lott, 2007). Organisms associated with late-onset infection include S. aureus, S. epidermidis, Pseudomonas and GBS.

Assessment of risk for newborn infection begins with a review of the maternal history and intrapartum record for evidence of maternal infection. Nurses should document maternal illness and infection during pregnancy on the prenatal record. Newborn assessment for clinical signs and laboratory analysis are important in diagnosis.

Laboratory Data

A complete blood count (CBC) with differential of white blood cell (WBC) components is the initial laboratory screening tool when sepsis is suspected. However, newer techniques, such as the polymerase chain reaction (PCR) test, may provide more accurate information. More than half of neonates actively infected may not produce enough bacterial growth to colonize and produce a positive blood culture (Brozanski, Jones, Krohn & Jordan, 2006). The use of intrapartal antibiotics may be one reason for these results. The DNA-based PCR test is used for bacterial, viral, protozoal and yeast infections, thus making detection of early-onset sepsis easier (Brozanski et al., 2006). Providers also should request a chest X-ray and C-reactive protein (Dear, 2005). Latex agglutination tests, serum interleukin, tumor necrosis factor (TNF-alpha), immunoelectrophoresis, acridine orange leukocyte cytospin test, and nitroblue tetrazolium (NBT) reduction are more specific tests to determine the causative agent (Dear, 2005).

Neonatal nurses often are responsible for collecting blood samples. Collection and handling methods can affect test results. Heelstick samples collected from unwarmed heels may give falsely high hematocrit (Hct) or hemoglobin results because of hemoconcentration. White cell counts are higher from unwarmed heel samples compared to venous and arterial samples and from specimens collected immediately after procedures that cause crying.

Neonatal nurses should consider mode of delivery when interpreting WBC and differentials. Consistency of sampling site and technique and allowing infants to rest 1 hour after procedures that cause crying are important.

Management

Essential elements of nursing care include recognition of newborns at risk and initial and ongoing assessment to facilitate early identification of infection. If separate teams are caring for the mother and newborn, communication between teams is imperative. Penicillin, ampicillin or amoxicillin, along with an aminoglycoside, is the initial treatment for a newborn with presumed primary sepsis. Primary sepsis is an infection that is not caused by a secondary condition, such as steroid use or another medical condition. If respiratory failure is present, providers can give surfactant (Dear, 2005). More research is needed before immunoglobulins, granulocyte colony-stimulating factor and granulocyte-macrophage colony-stimulating factor (GM-CSF) are used as routine adjunctive therapy.

Whether perinatal or intrapartal prophylaxis is used, discharge teaching must include written information regarding early signs of infant illness. The neonatal nurse should confirm that the infant has a primary pediatric provider whom the family can access after discharge.

GBS

According to the CDC (2002), GBS is a gram-positive, anaerobic bacterium that colonizes in the vagina or rectum of 10 percent to 30 percent of pregnant women. It is the most common cause of neonatal sepsis and meningitis in the United States. One percent to 2 percent of neonates born to women with GBS develop early-onset, invasive GBS disease. Early-onset, invasive GBS disease accounts for approximately 80 percent of all neonatal GBS infections, with a mortality rate of 5 percent to 20 percent.

There are seven GBS serotypes (Ia, Ib, Ic, II, III, IV and V), with III being the causative agent in almost all neonatal GBS infections, including early- and late-onset and meningitis (Blackburn, 2007). Maternal transmission occurs during labor and delivery through direct contact with contaminated secretions or through environmental exposure. Term newborns receive some passive immunity transplacentally when their mothers have type-specific IgG antibody to GBS strains (Blackburn, 2007).

Risk Factors
Table 22 identifies risk factors for GBS.

Table 22. Risk Factors for GBS	
Maternal	• Preterm labor • Heavy colonization • Prolonged rupture of membranes (>24 hours) • Intrapartum fever • Previous child with invasive GBS disease
Neonatal	• Prematurity • LBW • Heavy surface colonization

Clinical Signs
Newborn clinical signs may present rapidly, with some symptoms occurring within 4 to 6 hours and most within 24 hours of life. Early clinical signs may be subtle and nonspecific, making the maternal perinatal history important information in anticipating risk. Table 23 identifies clinical signs of GBS.

Table 23. Clinical Signs of GBS
• Changes in behavior (less responsive, floppy, irritable) • Gastrointestinal disturbances (poor feeding or vomiting) • Temperature instability • Jaundice • Apnea • Bradycardia • Tachypnea • Tachycardia • Pallor • Slowed capillary refill • Petechiae
Dear, 2005

Screening and Diagnosis

Antepartum screening and use of prophylactic antibiotics are controversial. The controversy focuses on the concern that using prophylactic antibiotics may increase the incidence of resistant bacterial infections. Table 24 identifies recommendations from the CDC (2002) consensus statement on screening and management.

Table 24. CDC Recommendations for GBS Screening and Management
• Universal prenatal screening of all pregnant women from 27 to 35 weeks gestation for vaginal and rectal GBS colonization • An approved regimen followed for women with sensitivity to penicillin • Antimicrobial susceptibility testing as part of the screening process • Routine intrapartum antibiotic prophylaxis for GBS colonization not recommended for women who are having planned cesarean deliveries, who have not begun labor or who have had a rupture of membrane • Use of an evidence-based algorithm for management of women with threatened preterm delivery • Use of an evidence-based algorithm for newborn management of exposure to intrapartum antibiotic prophylaxis
CDC, 2002

Management

When GBS is identified as the causative agent, providers can give benzylpenicillin or ampicillin (Dear, 2005). When the GBS-positive mother has received intrapartum antibiotic prophylaxis and labor and birth have been uneventful, the newborn may require no special diagnostic evaluation or treatment. There are no recommended special precautions regarding isolation for GBS, except in the case of a nursery outbreak.

E. coli

E. coli is a gram-negative rod that makes up most typical human fecal flora. It is the second most common cause of neonatal sepsis and meningitis in the United States (Dear, 2005).

Risk Factors

Risk for E. coli is by contamination of the birth canal with normal maternal gastrointestinal flora containing E. coli. Transmission is usually from mother to infant during labor and birth, when the infant comes in contact with contaminated birth-canal secretions.

Clinical Signs

Clinical signs of E. coli are essentially the same as for GBS. Early signs are subtle and nonspecific, but they can progress to elevated temperature, temperature instability, apnea and bradycardia, tachypnea, tachycardia, pallor, behavioral changes, gastrointestinal disturbances and poor feeding.

Screening and Diagnosis

Screening and diagnosis is made on a positive blood or tissue culture.

Management

Treatment involves use of an aminoglycoside alone or with cefotaxime if meningitis is suspected (Dear, 2005).

Tuberculosis

Tuberculosis (TB) is caused by the organism Mycobacterium tuberculosis. The incidence of TB in the United States has resurged since the late 1980s, in association with the HIV epidemic and society's mobility. The increase in HIV-infected women of childbearing age, coupled with an increase in the incidence of TB in non-White women, creates the potential for more pregnant women to be infected with TB and transmit the infection to their infants (CDC, 2006c, 2006d).

Congenital TB is rare, but possible. Transmission occurs by three routes: (1) from an infected placenta through the umbilical vein, (2) by ingestion of infected amniotic fluid or (3) by inhalation of infected amniotic fluid. Neonates can acquire TB through inhalation or ingestion of infected droplets, ingestion of infected breastmilk or contamination of traumatized skin or mucous membranes. Epidemiologically, congenital and neonatal TB is important; however, congenital and early neonatal TB have nearly the same presentation, treatment and prognosis.

Risk Factors
Table 25 identifies risk factors for TB.

Table 25. Risk Factors for TB
The incidence of TB is highest in urban, low-income areas and increases in the following groups: • Foreign-born persons • Migrant workers • First-generation immigrants from high-risk countries • African-Americans, Hispanics, Asians, American Indians and Alaskan natives • Homeless individuals or those residing in a shelter • Individuals with recent close contact with an infected person • IV-drug users • HIV-positive persons

Clinical Signs
Affected newborns are often born prematurely. Clinical manifestations are non-specific (Table 26). Onset of signs and symptoms usually occurs in the first 2 months, usually at 2 to 4 weeks.

Table 26. Clinical Manifestations of TB
• Respiratory distress • Fever • Poor feeding • Failure to thrive • Lethargy • Irritability • Hepatosplenomegaly

Screening and Diagnosis
The Mantoux Purified Protein Derivative (PPD) skin test usually is positive once the infant develops antibodies to the bacilli. Bacilli may be found in gastric aspirate, even when the PPD is nonreactive.

Management
Pregnant women diagnosed with active TB during pregnancy are treated with a 9-month regimen of isoniazid (INH) and rifampin. INH crosses the placenta; however, there is no evidence that it causes any risk to the fetus. There is no reported increased incidence of congenital defects in infants born to women who received rifampin during pregnancy (Kenner & Lott, 2007). Management

includes protecting an infant from contracting TB from a mother with active or inadequately treated infection. Table 27 lists appropriate interventions.

Table 27. Nursing Interventions to Prevent Maternal-newborn Transmission of TB
• Bathe the newborn to remove potentially infectious amniotic fluid. • Maintain strict standard precautions. • Separate the baby from the mother until maternal sputum cultures are negative. • Treat the infant prophylactically with INH and rifampin according to current protocols (Kenner & Lott, 2007). • Educate the mother and family about TB, its transmission and treatment; emphasize the importance of fully completing treatment. • Skin-test household contacts; if necessary obtain X-rays and a physical exam. • Follow-up with a primary pediatric provider in coordination with public health intervention.

Infants are at minimal risk and require no antituberculous treatment if they are born to mothers who have completed treatment for TB and have no evidence of disease. If the mother is being treated for TB at the time of delivery, the nurse should carefully evaluate the newborn. If no signs of congenital TB are present, the newborn should be placed on prophylactic INH until either the mother has a negative sputum smear and is known to be complying with treatment, or the infant is about 9 months old (Merck, 2005). Providers should skin test the newborn at birth and again at 3 months and 6 months if asymptomatic; the skin test should be repeated at 12 months after the INH has been stopped (Merck, 2005). Table 28 identifies treatment for infants positive for TB.

INH is secreted in breastmilk; however, no adverse effects on breastfeeding infants have been reported. Transfer of the drug to the infant may be decreased if the mother nurses or pumps just before taking her own daily dose of medication in the evening and if she substitutes a bottle for night feedings.

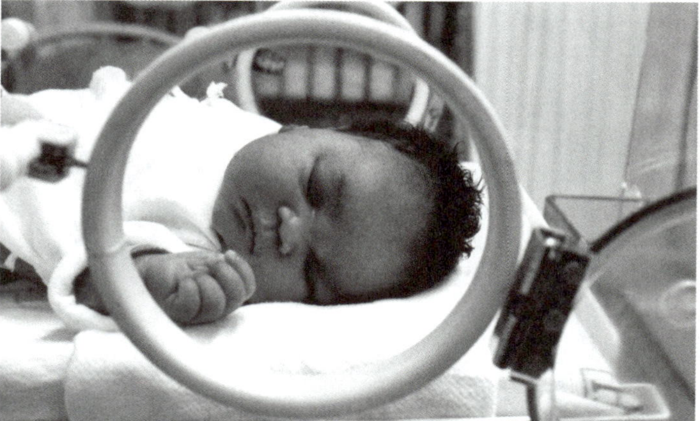

Table 28. Treatment of Infants with TB	
Standard therapy	• INH 10 mg/kg to15 mg/kg PO once per day for 10 months • Rifampin 10 mg/kg to 20 mg/kg PO once per day for 10 months • Pyrazinamide 20 mg/kg to 40 mg/kg PO **once per day for 10 months** AND • Streptomycin 20 mg/kg to 40 mg/kg intramuscular (IM) once per day for 2 months
Alternative therapy	INH and rifampin twice weekly for 10 months after the first 2 months of standard therapy
If breastfed	Pyridoxine supplementation
If streptomycin-resistant	Substitute with capreomycin or kanamycin
If CNS involvement	Prednisone 1 mg/kg PO once per day for 6 weeks to 8 weeks
When meningitis is no longer present	INH and rifampin for 10 months with steroids
Merck, 2005	

STIs

STIs affect approximately 19 million Americans every year (Cates, 1999) and can cause serious pregnancy complications. CDC (2006b) suggests gathering information from clients about STIs using the Five P's (Table 29). When using the Five P's with a pregnant woman, the provider asks her about the number of sexual partners she has had; if she uses condoms or other methods to prevent pregnancy and STIs; forms of sexual activity she has engaged in, such as oral, anal or vaginal sex; and her past history of STIs, including treatment and dates.

Table 29. The Five P's
1. Partners
2. Prevention of pregnancy
3. Protection from STIs
4. Practices
5. Past history of STIs

> **STIs affect approximately 19 million Americans every year and can cause serious pregnancy complications.**

Congenital Syphilis

Syphilis is caused by the spirochete Treponema pallidum. There are two modes of transmission: across the placenta and through direct contact with active genital lesions during vaginal delivery. At any stage of the disease, maternal syphilis can be transmitted to the fetus. Untreated secondary stage in the mother presents the greatest risk for transmission (almost 100 percent) and damage to the fetus, especially if it occurs during the period of organogenesis (Kenner & Lott, 2007).

Syphilis during pregnancy can cause preterm labor, PROM, stillbirth, congenital infection and neonatal death. All pregnant women should be tested for syphilis at their first prenatal visit (CDC, 2006c).

Neonates born to mothers with late, untreated syphilis usually present with no clinical signs (Dear, 2005). When the infection is acquired transplacentally, newborns may have signs of secondary syphilis with involvement of major organ systems, or they may only appear as LBW, premature infants.

Risk Factors
Table 30 identifies risk factors for congenital syphilis in the newborn.

Table 30. Risk Factors for Congenital Syphilis
• The mother has untreated syphilis.
• The mother's treatment is not well documented.
• There is evidence of maternal reinfection.
• The mother's treatment included non-penicillin drugs.
• The mother is HIV-positive.
• The mother receives treatment within 1 month of delivery.
• Maternal titers are unknown, have stayed the same or do not decrease with treatment.
• There is maternal history of substance abuse.

Clinical Signs
Table 31 identifies clinical signs of newborn syphilis.

Table 31. Clinical Signs of Newborn Syphilis
• Hepatosplenomegaly
• Jaundice
• Lymphadenopathy
• IUGR
• Failure to thrive
• Anemia
• Osteochondritis
• Vesicular bullous eruptions most commonly seen on palms of the hands and soles of the feet
• Rhinitis or snuffles
• Pulmonary abscesses
Dear, 2005

Screening and Diagnosis
Evaluation for congenital syphilis includes physical examination and serologic testing. Two types of serologic tests are used: nontreponemal and treponemal (Dear, 2005). Nontreponemal tests commonly used to screen newborns are the Venereal Disease Research Laboratory (VDRL) slide test and the rapid plasma reagin (RPR) test. These tests measure quantitative antibody levels, which are helpful indicators of disease activity and useful in assessing the adequacy of therapy. Infants born to positive mothers should receive quantitative tests (CDC, 2006c). Neonatal serum is preferred over cord blood for testing as cord blood can produce false-positive and

false-negative results because of transplacental transfer of maternal IgG antibody (Dear, 2005).

Treponemal tests include the fluorescent treponemal antibody absorption (FTA-ABS) test and the microhemagglutination test for T. pallidum (MHA-TP). These tests are used to establish a provisional diagnosis. Positive FTA-ABS and MHA-TP tests usually remain reactive for life. In a newborn with clinical findings suggestive of congenital syphilis, a positive VDRL and/or FTA-ABS test on serum provides strong evidence of congenital syphilis (Dear, 2005).

Providers should examine cerebrospinal fluid (CSF) VDRL in all infants born to mothers with syphilis during pregnancy and in those with suspected or proven congenital syphilis (Dear, 2005). Results of a CSF VDRL test, however, can be positive in an uninfected newborn with a transplacentally acquired, high-serum VDRL titer. Long-bone x-rays are not indicated if diagnosis has been established by other tests. Testing for antitreponemal immunoglobulin M (IgM) antibody, if available, may be included in the evaluation.

Management
The drug of choice for treatment of syphilis at any stage is parenteral penicillin G or benzylpenicillin (CDC, 2006c). Recommendations and duration of treatment for newborns vary depending on clinical status and serologic indicators.

In addition to standard precautions, transmission-based precautions are indicated for newborns with suspected or proven congenital syphilis until antibiotic therapy has been administered for a minimum of 24 hours. Breastfeeding is not contraindicated for infants whose mothers have been treated. Maternal education regarding effective treatment and long-term outcome is appropriate. Postdischarge follow-up for infected mothers and infants is imperative to ensure adequate treatment. Nurses should notify public health authorities for tracking and follow-up. Before discharge, nurses should confirm that mother and infant have a primary care provider and inform the mother about the need for serologic and other follow-up tests.

Gonorrhea
The causative organism for gonococcal infection in the neonate is Neisseria gonorrhoeae, gram-negative diplococci. Intrapartum contamination of the newborn usually occurs during contact with maternal secretions in the birth canal. However, it also can occur in utero after rupture of the membranes.

Risk Factors
Table 32 identifies risk factors for gonorrhea in the newborn.

Table 32. Risk Factors for Gonorrhea in the Newborn
Newborns at risk for gonorrhea have mothers who: • Have active gonococcal infection at the time of birth • Have a history in the current pregnancy of gonococcal disease with unknown follow-up status • Received no prenatal care • Have multiple sexual partners • Are adolescents

Clinical Signs

The most common clinical manifestation in neonates is ophthalmia neonatorum or conjunctivitis (CDC, 2006c). Infection also may present as scalp abscesses (related to intrapartal scalp monitoring), vaginitis or systemic disease with bacteremia, meningitis and/or endocarditis (Kenner & Lott, 2007).

Screening and Diagnosis

Screening and diagnosis is done through blood and tissue cultures. If the organism *Neisseria gonorrhoeae* is identified, then the diagnosis is gonorrhea.

Management

Prevention of neonatal infection is the goal of management. Perinatal prevention strategies include routine screening of all pregnant women for gonorrhea at the first prenatal visit; a second culture late in the third trimester for women at high risk of exposure; and neonatal prophylactic instillation of 0.5 percent erythromycin, 1 percent tetracycline or 1 percent silver-nitrate eye drops immediately after birth (Kenner & Lott, 2007).

Correct administration of eye prophylaxis prevents gonococcal infection in most infants. Nurses should examine infants for clinical evidence of ophthalmia neonatorum (conjunctivitis), purulent discharge and corneal ulcerations, scalp abscess and signs of disseminated infection/sepsis. Cultures of eye discharge, blood and CSF can confirm diagnosis and determine antibiotic sensitivity. Single-dose Ceftriaxone is the recommended antimicrobial therapy for nondisseminated infections, including ophthalmia neonatorum, and for infants born to mothers with active gonorrhea at the time of delivery (Dear, 2005). In infants with hyperbilirubinemia, Cefotaxime in two divided doses for 7 days is an alternative. The eyes of infants with conjunctivitis should be irrigated with saline at birth and regularly until the discharge is cleared. Ophthalmic antibiotic ointment alone is not adequate for treatment and is not necessary when appropriate systemic antibiotic treatment is given (CDC, 2006c).

Newborns with gonococcal infection, including ophthalmia neonatorum, should be managed with transmission-based precautions in addition to standard precautions. Isolation should be maintained until appropriate antimicrobial therapy has been administered for 24 hours (Dear, 2005). There are no contraindications to breastfeeding with maternal gonococcal infection. Gonococcal infection must be reported to public health officials. In addition, communication with the primary pediatric provider facilitates follow-up for well-child care and ophthalmology.

Hepatitis B

Although five different types of hepatitis virus exist (A, B, C, D and E), hepatitis B virus (HBV) is the one seen most often in perinatal and neonatal infection. Hepatitis C virus (HCV) also is seen in the perinatal population, but transmission is relatively rare except in women with high viral titers and with human immunodeficiency virus (HIV) (CDC, 2006b, 2006c; Dear, 2005). Hepatitis E is a rising concern in developing countries (Dear, 2005).

Risk Factors
The rate of perinatal HBV transmission is high (76 percent) in mothers with acute HBV in the third trimester or near the time of delivery and low (10 percent) when HBV occurs in the first 2 trimesters (Dear, 2005). There is some genetic predisposition to HBV, as the presence of an "e" antigen HBeAg in maternal blood puts the infant at greater risk for infection. Ethnicity also is a factor. In a study in the United Kingdom (Dear, 2005), Chinese mothers were most often carriers, followed by African, Asian and Caucasian women.

Clinical Signs
Most infants born to women with HBV are asymptomatic at birth (CDC, 2006c). Ninety percent of infants born to women positive for both the hepatitis B surface antigen (HBsAG) and the hepatitis B envelop antigen (HBeAG) are at risk for developing HBV during the first year of life if not treated (Kenner & Lott, 2007).

Screening and Diagnosis
Neonatal infection usually occurs at birth when the infant comes in direct contact with contaminated maternal blood and vaginal fluid. Mothers positive for HBsAG are infectious, and those positive for HBeAg are highly infectious. Table 33 lists CDC (2006b) HBV screening guidelines for pregnant women. The Advisory Committee on Immunization Practices (ACIP) (2005) states that all pregnant women should be tested again when admitted for delivery and recommends that all adolescents and adults not previously immunized receive the hepatitis B immune globulin (HBIG) vaccine.

Table 33. Screening Guidelines for HBV in Pregnant Women

• Screen all pregnant women for HBsAG.
• Repeat HBsAG testing late in pregnancy for:
  – HBsAG-negative women at high risk of HBV (intravenous [IV] drug users and women with STIs)
  – Women who have clinical evidence of hepatitis

CDC, 2006b

Management
Prevention is the most appropriate course of action. For all infants born to women who are HBV-positive, ACIP (2005) recommends giving the first dose of the HBIG vaccine at birth. Subsequent doses are due at 1 month and 6 months (Pickering, 2006). All infants born to women who are not HBV-positive should receive three scheduled doses, with the first given at birth or before discharge, the second at 1 month to 2 months of age, and the last at 6 months to 18 months of age. Table 34 identifies the recommended immunization procedure.

Breastfeeding is not contraindicated as long as the infant receives the HBIG vaccine according to recommendations (ACIP, 2005).

Table 34. HBIG Dose and Administration
• The standard dose of HBIG is prophylaxis of infants born to hepatitis B surface antigen (HBsAg)-positive women and 0.06 mL/kg for all other applications. • HBIG may be administered simultaneously with hepatitis B vaccine but in a different injection site. • For infants, HBIG should be administered intramuscularly in the anterolateral thigh using a 22- to 25-gauge needle that is 7/8 inch to 1 inch in length (CDC, 2002). • Vaccination with certain live-virus vaccines (measles, mumps, rubella and varicella) should be deferred at least 3 months after administration of HBIG because HBIG can inhibit the response to these vaccines (CDC, 2002). • HBIG should be stored at 2 C to 8 C and should not be frozen.
ACIP, 2005

Nurses should document maternal screening information on the prenatal record and report positive test results to the health department. Nurses should be familiar with guidelines for prevention and prophylaxis for newborns of women who are HBsAg-positive or who have unknown HBV status. Table 35 identifies nursing interventions for infants of HBsAG-positive women.

Table 35. Nursing Interventions for Infants of HBsAG-positive Women
• Bathe infants after delivery to remove maternal blood and reduce risk of transmission. • Maintain strict standard precautions. • Educate mothers about HBV and the importance of a complete series of immunizations for their infants. • Provide written documentation on an immunization card with discharge instructions of the infant's perinatal HBV exposure, HBIG status and vaccine administration. • Notify the infant's primary care provider of the mother's HBsAg-positive status. • Educate breastfeeding mothers about reducing the chance of cracked nipples, which could cause additional exposure of the infant to maternal blood and serous fluids.

Case management and follow-up care are essential to ensure compliance with immunizations and assessment (ACIP, 2005). For infants whose mothers have hepatitis B, antibody testing after the vaccination series is necessary only to determine the presence of adequate levels of HBeAg and HBsAg (ACIP, 2005).

HIV

HIV is the virus that causes acquired immunodeficiency syndrome (AIDS). AIDS represents the most advanced stage of HIV infection. HIV infection is transmitted from mother to fetus in utero transplacentally, intrapartally through contact with maternal blood, and in breastmilk.

Risk Factors
Table 36 identifies HIV risk factors for women of childbearing age.

Table 36. HIV Risk Factors for Women of Childbearing Age
• Using IV drugs • Having multiple sex partners • Living in geographic areas with high HIV incidence rates • Being African-American or Hispanic • Having another STI
CDC, 2006b, c; Simpson, 2006

Clinical Signs
Neonates born to HIV-positive women are most often asymptomatic at birth. They usually develop signs and symptoms between 4 months and 6 months of age with an incubation of 6 weeks to 10 years (CDC, 2006b, 2006c). Table 37 identifies clinical manifestations of HIV and AIDS in infants and children.

Table 37. Clinical Manifestations of HIV and AIDS in Infants and Children
• Generalized lymphadenopathy • Hepatosplenomegaly • Failure to thrive • Oral and cutaneous candidiasis • Recurrent diarrhea • Recurrent invasive bacterial infections • Opportunistic infections
Kenner & Lott, 2007

Screening and Diagnosis
Perinatal transmission is difficult to diagnose by standard immunoassays (ELISA and Western blot). Maternal IgG antibodies in the fetus and newborn cause many infants born to HIV-infected mothers to test positive for HIV antibodies at birth. The actual status of these infants should be determined by serial HIV tests (AAP & ACOG, 2007). Maternal IgG antibodies can be detected in the infant up to 18 months after birth. With proper screening and antiretroviral prophylaxis during labor and after birth, the risk of vertical transmission rate decreases (AAP & ACOG, 2007; Simpson, 2006).

Determining an infant's HIV status has improved with the development of the polymerase chain reaction (PCR), HIV-p24 antigen and HIV cultures. The PCR detects the virus and not the antibody; therefore, it is not affected by persistent maternal antibody levels. The sensitivity of HIV-p24 antigen and HIV cultures is greater than the DNA/RNA PCR. RNA assays are more sensitive. Using these non-antibody-based tests, providers can diagnose most infected infants by 3 to 6 months of age. Infants tend to have higher viral loads than older children and adults and progress to AIDs faster (Sundaravaradan et al., 2006). Infants at risk for HIV should be tested at birth to 2 weeks, at 1 to 2 months, and at 3 to 6 months (AIDS Education and Training Center [AETC], 2006). Table 38 provides some of CDC's HIV screening recommendations for pregnant women.

Table 38. CDC HIV Screening Recommendations for Pregnant Women
• HIV screening should be included in the routine panel of prenatal screening tests for all pregnant women. • HIV screening is recommended after the patient is notified that testing will be performed unless the patient declines (opt-out screening). • Separate written consent for HIV testing should not be required; general consent for medical care should be considered sufficient to encompass consent for HIV testing. • Repeat screening in the third trimester is recommended in certain jurisdictions with elevated rates of HIV infection among pregnant women.
CDC, 2006c

Management

HIV prevention is the ultimate goal. Research into pharmacological prevention in the neonate is promising, with clinical trials examining combinations of antiretroviral agents. Combinations include zidovudine (ZDV) with nevirapine (NVP), nelfinavir (NFV) and lamivudine (3TC) given within 48 hours of birth and for the first 6 weeks of life (National Institute of Child Health and Human Development [NICHD] & National Institute of Allergy and Infectious Diseases [NIAID], 2006). Table 39 identifies nursing considerations for newborns with HIV.

Table 39. Management of Newborns with HIV
• Strict adherence to standard precautions • Bathing the infant as soon as possible after birth to minimize exposure to maternal blood and body fluids • Breastfeeding as a contraindication to transmission via breastmilk in developed countries • Maternal and family education about HIV infection and treatment • Confirmation of a primary pediatric provider and referral to a center for HIV follow-up and treatment • Linking the family to support services • Treatment based on clinical manifestations of the disease
Kenner & Lott, 2007

Chlamydia

Chlamydia is the most widespread STI in the United States (Kenner & Lott, 2007). *Chlamydia trachomatis* is the bacterial agent most commonly found in perinatal infection (CDC, 2006c; Kenner & Lott, 2007). Transmission occurs at birth when the infant comes in contact with contaminated vaginal fluids in the birth canal.

Risk Factors

Women age 20 and younger are most strongly associated with chlamydial infections. The prevalence of chlamydia is higher among Black and economically disadvantaged persons (Darville, 2006). Acquisition occurs in approximately 50 percent of infants born vaginally to infected mothers and in some infants delivered by cesarean with intact membranes (Kenner & Lott, 2007).

Clinical Signs
The principal clinical manifestations in infants are conjunctivitis and pneumonia. Conjuctivitis usually appears within 4 to 14 days after birth. Clinical symptoms include swelling of one or both eyelids and micropurulent discharge. Chronic infection can cause conjunctival scarring, adhesions of the eyelid and corneal scarring; loss of vision is rare (Kenner & Lott, 2007). Afebrile pneumonia typically occurs at 6 to 8 weeks of age.

Screening and Diagnosis
Diagnosis is from laboratory tests. A conjunctival scraping and smear are made for Giemsa staining. Direct immunofluorescent antibody staining or enzyme immunoassay should be done to confirm the diagnosis.

Management
Topical eye treatment consists of sulfacetamide or tetracycline drops or ointment for 3 weeks. Systemic therapy with oral erythromycin estolate or erythromycin ethylsuccinate for 3 weeks often is needed to eradicate the organism from the respiratory tract. Breastfeeding is permitted unless antibiotics used to treat maternal infection are contraindicated (Kenner & Lott, 2007).

Herpes Simplex
There are two types of herpes simplex viruses, HSV-1 and HSV-2. HSV-1 usually is transmitted horizontally via contact with oral lesions, fever blisters or cold sores. HSV-2, often called genital herpes, involves the genitals and usually is transmitted via sexual contact (CDC, 2006c). HSV-2 is the most common cause of disease in the newborn; however, HSV-1 accounts for 15 percent to 20 percent of all genital herpes simplex infections and does cause HSV disease in the newborn (Kenner & Lott, 2007). Either type can occur almost anywhere in the body. HSV-1 is more closely associated with herpes found outside the genital area.

Transmission usually occurs intrapartally with ascending infection after rupture of membranes or through contact with an infected birth canal during vaginal delivery. Postnatal transmission from mother and father to newborn, including transmission by breastfeeding in the presence of breast lesions, has been documented (Kenner & Lott, 2007).

Risk Factors
Risk factors for transmission of HSV infection from mother to fetus/newborn include ruptured membranes, intrauterine fetal monitoring and fetal scalp sampling; the risk of contracting the disease is higher if the mother is experiencing a primary infection (30 percent to 50 percent incidence) as opposed to a recurrent outbreak (<5 percent) (Kenner & Lott, 2007). Knowledge of maternal HSV status is vital in minimizing transmission and identifying infants at risk.

Clinical Signs
HSV infection is associated with an increased incidence of prematurity and LBW. Clinical signs may or may not be present at birth and can take as long as 3 weeks to manifest. Symptoms are nonspecific and similar to those of bacterial sepsis; therefore, providers must obtain a thorough history when trying to decide on a course of action.

> **HSV-2 is the most common cause of disease in the newborn.**

Screening and Diagnosis
Laboratory tests can differentiate HSV infection from other bacterial and viral infections. Routine cultures should be obtained from vesicles on the skin, oropharyngeal or eye secretions, or stool. Viral typing is done for epidemiologic purposes only.

Management
To optimize outcome and decrease sequelae and supportive therapy, treatment includes antiviral pharmacologic intervention with acyclovir and vidarabine. There is no cure; once infected, the virus remains in the host forever with the possibility of subsequent reactivations. Long-term prognosis is good for infants whose infection is localized to the skin, eyes or mouth, but poor for infants with systemic disease. Table 40 identifies nursing responsibilities for treating a family with HSV.

Table 40. Nursing Responsibilities for Treating a Family with HSV
• Careful history-taking about maternal and family HSV status
• Thorough examination and ongoing assessment of the newborn
• Maternal and family education regarding transmission and prevention, including careful hand-washing before handling the infant
• Instruction to the parent with an oral lesion about wearing a mask and refraining from kissing the infant until lesions have crusted and dried
• Isolation of neonates with HSV infection or with positive cultures in the absence of disease
• Instruction to the mother that breastfeeding is permitted as long as there are no lesions present on the breasts
Kenner & Lott, 2007

TORCH Infections

TORCH infections are a group of infections that if acquired by a pregnant woman can lead to birth defects. TORCH is an acronym for **t**oxoplasmosis, **o**ther infections, **r**ubella, CMV and **h**erpes.

Toxoplasmosis
The causative agent of toxoplasmosis is a protozoan parasite called Toxoplasma gondii. Human infection occurs after eating undercooked meat containing the cysts of toxoplasma or handling soil or cat litter infested with the oocytes of the organism. It is transmitted perinatally via placental colonization from the mother to the fetus; the infection only occurs if the mother acquires the primary infection while pregnant. Intrauterine transmission rates rise with increasing gestational age, from 10 percent in the first trimester to 90 percent in the third (Pickering, 2006). Fetal and neonatal morbidity and mortality increase with earlier transmission. Maternal infection after 24 weeks gestation usually results in mild effects on the fetus and newborn. Ninety percent of infected infants are asymptomatic at birth but develop symptoms within the first 2 months of life. (Pickering, 2006). Clinical signs and symptoms in the newborn include the classic triad of chorioretinitis, hydrocephalus and intracranial calcifications, accompanied by seizures, hepatosplenomegaly, late-onset jaundice, rash and petechiae secondary to thrombocytopenia. Symptomatic and seropositive asymptomatic infants should be treated. No additional isolation precautions are recommended (Pickering, 2006). Breastfeeding is not discouraged unless antibiotics used in treatment are contraindicated.

Other Infections
For TORCH infection, "other" generally refers to hepatitis B, syphilis and herpes zoster.

Rubella
Rubella, or German measles, is a viral infection that can be transmitted through nasopharyngeal secretions or across the placenta. Immunization has significantly reduced the incidence; however, approximately 10 percent of young adults are susceptible to rubella (Cooper & Alford, 2006), creating the potential for congenital infection. Congenital defects after maternal infection vary widely depending on the timing of exposure. Because most defects are associated with infection during the first trimester, rubella titers are drawn on all pregnant women during this period. Table 41 identifies the most common clinical manifestations of congenital rubella. Systemic infection often presents with purple lesions called blueberry muffin rash.

Table 41. Clinical Manifestations of Congenital Rubella
• Cataracts
• Heart disease (PDA or septal defects)
• Neurological problems
• Deafness
• LBW

Prevention via immunization is the best management; treatment for active infection is supportive. Transmission-based and standard precautions are recommended for congenitally infected infants. Infants with congenital infection shed virus in nasopharyngeal secretions and urine for 1 year or longer and are contagious unless cultures after 3 months of age are negative. Breastfeeding is permissible after the infectious stage has passed in the mother.

CMV
CMV, a member of the herpes family, is the most frequent cause of congenital viral infections in humans (Kenner & Lott, 2007). Perinatal transmission is vertical through the birth canal or across the placenta; CMV also may be passed through breastmilk. In utero, transmission can occur if the mother has a primary infection or reactivation during pregnancy. Horizontal transmission can occur with exposure to infectious secretions.

Almost all newborns with congenital CMV infection are asymptomatic. Table 42 lists clinical manifestations in symptomatic neonates. Most congenitally infected infants appear normal at birth but develop signs later in life; the most common signs are progressive sensorineural hearing loss, mental retardation and developmental delays. Infected infants shed virus in saliva for 2 to 4 years and in urine for up to 6 years or longer, with the highest quantities of virus excreted in the first 6 months.

Table 42. Clinical Manifestations of CMV in Symptomatic Neonates
• Petechiae
• Microcephaly
• Hepatosplenomegaly
• Jaundice
• IUGR
• Chorioretinitis
• Intracranial calcifications
Kenner & Lott, 2007

CMV is neither preventable nor treatable. Breastfeeding is contraindicated for seropositive mothers unless the infant is also seropositive. Parent education regarding CMV infection, viral shedding and outcome is appropriate.

Developmental and audiologic follow-up are important considerations of discharge planning for these infants.

Herpes
See herpes discussion beginning on page 85.

Vitamin K Deficiency

One in 200 to 1 in 400 newborns not treated prophylactically with vitamin K at birth develop hemorrhagic disease of the newborn (HDN) (Blackburn, 2007). Hemorrhage occurs as a result of hypoprothrombinemia due to deficiencies in vitamin K-dependent coagulation factors. Table 43 identifies causes of deficiencies in various vitamin K-dependent coagulation factors (II, VII, IX, X).

In the past, providers classified HDN as early, classic and late. Two classifications are now used: early and late vitamin K deficiency bleeding (VKDB). Table 44 identifies characteristics of both classifications. Onset of bleeding in the first 24 hours of life is rare and life threatening; it usually is associated with maternal drugs (warfarin, anticonvulsants, antituberculous chemotherapy), but it can be idiopathic in origin (Blackburn, 2007).

> **One in 200 to 1 in 400 newborns not treated prophylactically with vitamin K at birth develop HDN.**

Table 43. Causes of Deficiencies in Vitamin K-dependent Coagulation Factors (II, VII, IX, X)
• Poor placental transport of vitamin K
• Lack of intestinal colonization by bacteria known to synthesize vitamin K
• Maternal use of anticoagulants, anticonvulsants and antibiotics
• Exclusive breastfeeding
• History of prenatal asphyxia
Blackburn, 2007

Table 44. Characteristics of Early and Late VKDB		
	Early VKDB	**Late VKDB**
Onset	Birth to 2 weeks	2 to 12 weeks
Affected infants	Breastfed infants who develop hypoprothrombinemia secondary to vitamin K deficiency	• Breastfed infants who have not received vitamin K prophylaxis • Infants with gastrointestinal disorders associated with significant fat malabsorption (e.g., cystic fibrosis, biliary atresia)
Signs	• Generalized ecchymosis • Gastrointestinal bleeding • Bleeding from the circumcision site or umbilical cord; oozing from puncture sites (Blackburn, 2003)	• Generalized ecchymosis • Gastrointestinal bleeding • Bleeding from the circumcision site or umbilical cord; oozing from puncture sites (Blackburn, 2003)
Treatment	Parenteral vitamin K (AAP Committee on the Fetus and Newborn, 2006)	Parenteral vitamin K (AAP Committee on the Fetus and Newborn, 2006)

Laboratory diagnosis of vitamin K deficiency has traditionally relied on the indirect measurement of various vitamin K-dependent coagulation proteins. Findings include prolonged prothrombin time (PT) and partial thromboplastin time (PTT) (Blackburn, 2007). Interpretation of these studies is complicated because expected coagulation factors in the newborn are 30 percent to 60 percent of adult levels, making PT prolonged in the newborn when compared with an adult. One-stage PT is significantly increased only in instances of severe deficiency.

Puckett and Offringa (2006) coauthored a Cochrane Review examining prophylactic vitamin K for neonatal deficiency and found that a single dose of vitamin K prevents the classic form of vitamin K deficiency. The AAP Committee on Fetus and Newborn (2006) recommends that every neonate receive a single intramuscular dose of 0.5 mg to 1.0 mg of prophylactic vitamin K1 oxide (phytonadione) at birth for prevention of early VKDB; parenteral vitamin K is required for late VKDB. The link between parenteral vitamin K and childhood cancer has not been supported, and oral forms of vitamin K, especially for the treatment of late VKDB, need further research (AAP Committee on Fetus and Newborn, 2006). Table 45 identifies nursing considerations when administering vitamin K.

Table 45. Nursing Considerations for Administering Vitamin K

• Give vitamin K as an intramuscular injection in the vastus lateralis muscle using a 25-guage, 5/8-inch needle.
  – Give a one-time-only prophylactic dose of 0.5 mg to 1.0 mg in the delivery room or upon admission to the nursery.
  – Give an additional dose 6 to 8 hours later if the mother received anticoagulant therapy during pregnancy.
• Observe for pain and edema at the injection site.
• Observe for bleeding from the umbilical cord, circumcision site, nose and gastrointestinal tract; this is typically evident on the second or third day if it occurs.
• Check that follow-up labs are ordered.
• Give vitamin K before any invasive procedure (circumcision, spinal tap).
• Keep vitamin K away from direct light.

Neonatal Polycythemia

Neonatal polycythemia is a venous Hct of >65 percent or 22 g/dL (Blackburn, 2007). Evidence of polycythemia usually presents within the first 48 to 72 hours of life.

Risk Factors
Table 46 identifies risk factors for neonatal polycythemia.

Clinical Signs
Newborns with polycythemia are usually plethoric (ruddy) in appearance and may be otherwise asymptomatic. Increased blood viscosity is the underlying mechanism responsible for clinically significant polycythemia. Hyperviscosity impairs peripheral blood flow, causing sluggish circulation. Eventually, capillary circulation throughout the body is affected, compromising various organ systems (Figure 4).

Table 46. Risk Factors for Polycythemia

- Twin-to-twin transfusion, maternal-fetal transfusion and delayed cord clamping, resulting in increased fetal-blood volume
- Placenta infarction, placenta previa, TORCH and other viral infections, and postmaturity, resulting in uteroplacental insufficiency and increased production of red blood cells
- Genetic disorders, such as trisomy 21, 13 and 18, and Beckwith-Weidemann syndrome
- In utero stress, chronic hypoxia-IUGR, cyanotic heart disease (Blackburn, 2007)
- Mothers with diabetes, chronic hypertension or who smoke or abuse substances (Blackburn, 2007)
- Born at high altitudes (Blackburn, 2007)
- Increased red blood cell production or red cell transfusion

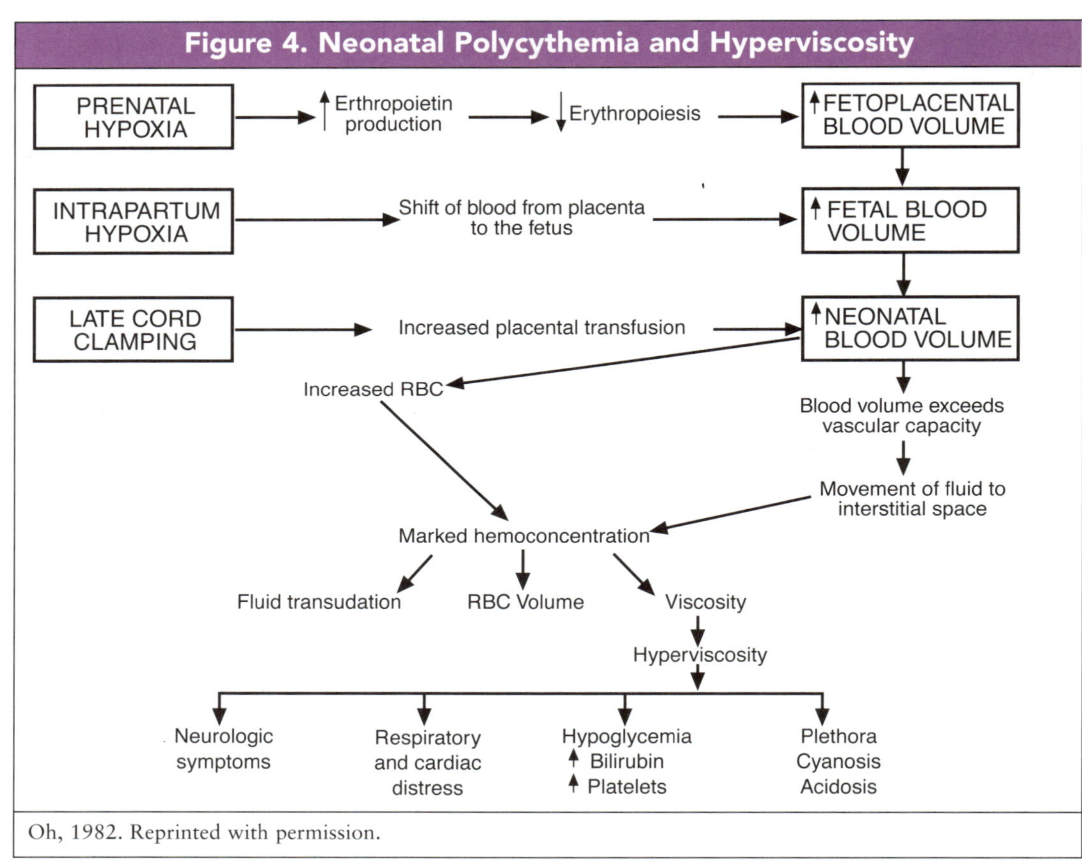

Figure 4. Neonatal Polycythemia and Hyperviscosity

Oh, 1982. Reprinted with permission.

Common CNS signs include lethargy, poor feeding, tremors and jitteriness; seizures and cerebrovascular accidents are rare (Lessaris, 2005). Hypoglycemia is the most common metabolic complication found in polycythemia, however, hypocalcemia also is seen. Hyperbilirubinemia associated with polycythemia is caused by destruction of excessive RBCs. Cardiopulmonary findings include tachypnea, cyanosis and tachycardia. Pulmonary circulatory compromise can cause pulmonary hypertension, retained lung fluid and respiratory distress. Hyperviscosity also can affect the kidneys, causing renal vein thrombosis and renal failure, and the gastrointestinal tract, leading to necrotizing enterocolitis in term newborns (Lessaris, 2005).

Screening and Diagnosis

A screening Hct before 6 hours of age helps detect polycythemia and allows for appropriate management. The average Hct for term newborns on the first postnatal day of life is 61 percent; the peak value occurs at 2 hours of age, followed by a progressive decrease through the first 24 hours (Lessaris, 2005). The initial rise in HcT is due to the movement of fluid out of the intravascular space.

Sampling site affects Hct values in the newborn. Capillary Hct (from heel sticks) are higher than venous values, especially during the early transition period when peripheral perfusion is sluggish. Nurses should analyze a venous Hct when a high screening capillary Hct is detected.

Management

The management goal is to reduce the central venous Hct to <65 percent in symptomatic newborns. Generally, if the Hct is between 65 percent and 75 percent, increasing fluids, especially if dehydration is present, and monitoring Hct, glucose and symptoms of polycythemia are appropriate. If the Hct is >65 percent, then a partial exchange transfusion may be necessary. If several testings confirm that the Hct is >75 percent, then a partial exchange transfusion may be used (Lessaris, 2005). Monitoring the Hct and glucose levels is essential whether or not the infant is treated. If the infant is symptomatic, then the cause of this problem is important. Treating the symptoms does not resolve the underlying problem. Treatment of asymptomatic newborns is controversial. The newborn should be kept hydrated, and blood glucose and calcium levels should be monitored.

Jaundice

In the United States each year, more than half of all full-term newborns become clinically jaundiced (Hansen, 2006). Jaundice is yellow skin pigmentation caused by increased levels of unconjugated bilirubin. For most, jaundice causes no problems. However, some infants have problems when jaundice is complicated by dehydration, prematurity, difficult delivery or other reasons. Nurses should understand bilirubin metabolism and hyperbilirubinemia, know how to recognize newborns at risk for developing hyperbilirubinemia, and be able to assess infants for early detection of jaundice.

The terms physiologic jaundice, pathologic jaundice and hyperbilirubinemia sometimes are used interchangeably. With inconsistent terminology and definitions, the understanding of jaundice becomes more difficult (Blackburn, 2007). Table 47 provides a list of terms and definitions.

Bilirubin Metabolism

Conjugated or direct bilirubin is bilirubin that has been metabolized or conjugated by the liver. It is water soluble and passes from the liver through the common bile duct to the intestines for excretion. Most direct bilirubin is excreted in the stool. Some is reabsorbed in the colon and excreted in urine via the enterohepatic circulation. Unconjugated or indirect bilirubin is bilirubin that has not been metabolized by the liver. It is fat soluble and not easily excreted in stool or urine. It poses the greatest risk for newborns. Excessive accumulation of unconjugated bilirubin causes deposition in the skin, causing jaundice in the brain, where it can be toxic and lead to acute bilirubin encephalopathy (ABE) (formerly known as kernicterus). In utero, most fetal bilirubin is unconjugated. It readily crosses the

> **In the United States each year, more than half of all full-term newborns become clinically jaundiced.**

Table 47. Jaundice Terms and Definitions

Term	Definition/Description
Hyperbilirubinemia	Jaundice that: • Occurs within the first 24 hours after birth OR • Lasts for more than 1 week in a term newborn OR • Has excessive bilirubin levels 　– Total bilirubin >12 mg/dL to 13 mg/dL 　OR 　– Direct bilirubin >1.5 mg/dL to 2 mg/dL 　OR 　– A rate of rise in bilirubin >5 mg/dL/day Hyperbilirubinemia is an increased bilirubin level that may be due to factors that can cause exaggerated physiologic jaundice or pathologic jaundice. It sometimes mistakenly is used as a synonym for pathologic jaundice. Blackburn, 2007.
Physiologic jaundice	An expected process that affects many term newborns. It usually is a transient, benign condition that appears in the first 2 to 3 days of life and resolves within 7 to 10 days. Bilirubin level is >5 mg/dL to 7 mg/dL (Blackburn, 2007) and rarely exceeds 15 mg/dL. It is caused by physiological processes, such as metabolism of red blood cells or increased bilirubin production from hemolysis of RBCs, decreased albumin binding capacity and functional immaturity of the newborn liver. Almost all newborns experience elevated bilirubin levels, but only half show observable signs. Incidence of physiologic jaundice differs markedly according to race. Infants of Asian, American Indian and Eskimo descent have a mean bilirubin level twice as high as White infants; Blacks have a lower incidence than Whites (AHRQ, 2002).
Pathologic jaundice	Caused by pathologic processes that change expected bilirubin metabolism, including conditions that increase hemoglobin destruction, increase reabsorption of bilirubin from the intestine, impair liver conjugation or interfere with liver excretion of conjugated bilirubin (Blackburn, 2007). Conditions that can cause increased hemoglobin destruction include maternal-fetal blood group incompatibility (Rh, ABO), increased hemoglobin load from cephalohematoma and polycythemia, neonatal sepsis and congenital RBC abnormalities. Bilirubin level is the same as for physiologic jaundice when there is hyperbilirubinemia. Other conditions that increase the risk of pathologic jaundice include: • Passage of the first stool later than 12 hours after birth, resulting in increased enterohepatic circulation • Drugs (morphine and phenobarbital) that compete with bilirubin for binding sites on albumin, raising the levels of free bilirubin • Births at high altitude that can result in increased bilirubin production, accompanied by delayed bilirubin clearance in response to decreased oxygen availability and increased RBC production • Asphyxia, hypoxia, hypothermia and hypoglycemia, all of which impair liver conjugation • Congenital conditions, such as biliary atresia and cystic fibrosis, that can cause hepatic obstruction

placenta and is excreted by the maternal liver. The newborn, therefore, is rarely born jaundiced.

Destruction of circulating RBCs accounts for approximately 75 percent of the bilirubin produced in the healthy term newborn (Blackburn, 2007). RBC destruction occurs in the reticuloendothelial system and is an expected process that gets rid of aging, immature or malformed cells.

Hemoglobin in the RBC is broken down into heme, globin and iron. Bilirubin is produced from the breakdown of heme-containing proteins (Blackburn, 2007). Enzymes convert the heme to biliverdin and then to unconjugated bilirubin. A healthy newborn produces on average twice as much bilirubin (6 mg/kg/day to 10 mg/kg/day) as an adult (3 mg/kg/day to 4 mg/kg/day) because of a higher concentration of circulating red cells, a shorter RBC life span (70 days to 90 days) and limited hepatic enzyme production (beta-glucuronidase) (Blackburn, 2007). Figure 5 depicts the four stages of bilirubin metabolism.

Figure 5. Four Stages of Bilirubin Metabolism

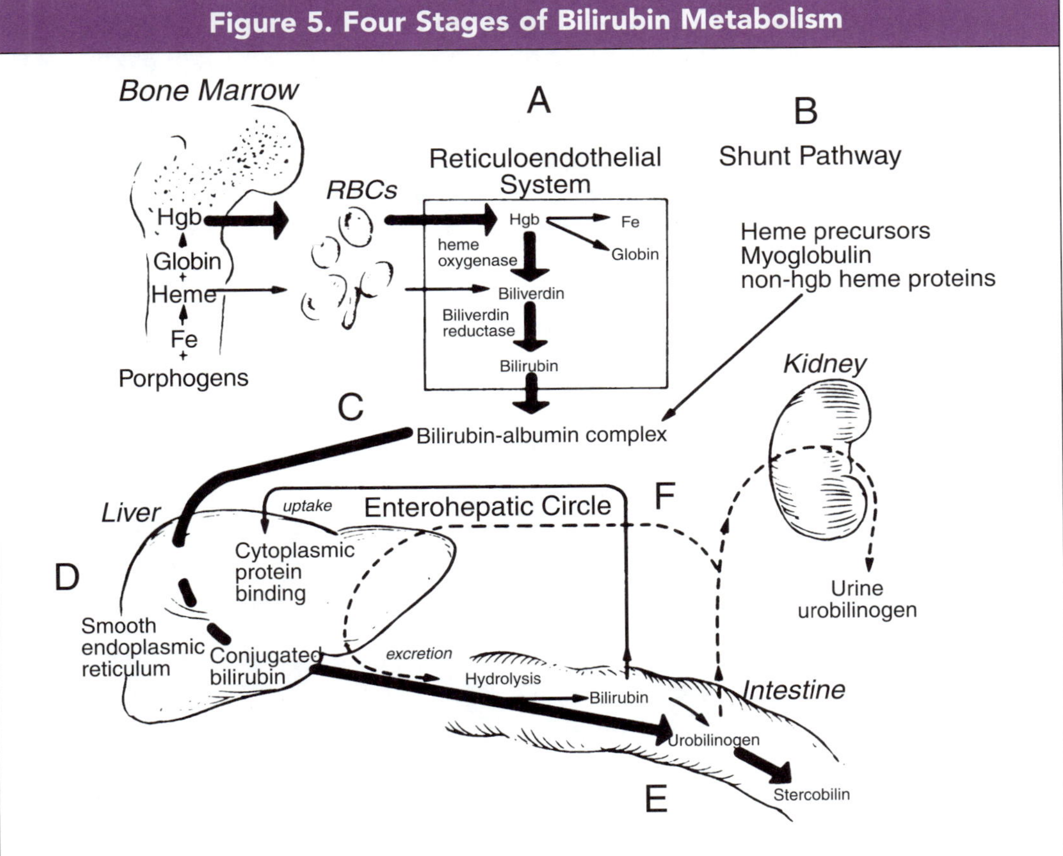

Production: (A) Hemoglobin is broken down into heme, iron and globin. Heme is further broken down by enzymes into biliverdin and then bilirubin (indirect). (B) Heme from nonhemoglobin sources is also converted into bilirubin. Transport: (C) Most bilirubin is carried in the blood to the liver bound to albumin; the rest is unbound or free. Conjugation: (D) The liver converts indirect bilirubin into water-soluble direct bilirubin, which it excretes into the intestine via the biliary tree. Excretion: (E) Direct bilirubin is converted in the intestines into urobilinogen and stercobilin. A small amount of urobilinogen may also be excreted in urine or returned to the bloodstream (- - - line). (F) Some urobilinogen is unconjugated by enzymes and converted back to indirect bilirubin. This indirect bilirubin is absorbed across the intestinal wall, reenters the circulation and returns to the liver (—line).

Gartner & Hollander, 1972. Reprinted with permission.

Bilirubin Conjugation

Unconjugated bilirubin is transported to the liver through the bilirubin-albumin complex. In the liver, unconjugated bilirubin and glucuronic acid combine in the presence of the enzyme glucoronyl transferase to form conjugated bilirubin glucuronide. This conjugated bilirubin passes through the common bile duct and into the intestine, where it is reduced by bacteria and excreted. Reduced hepatic enzyme activity and reduced albumin binding capacity predispose the newborn to decreased capacity for bilirubin conjugation. Bilirubin that is not bound to albumin is called free or unbound bilirubin. The amount of free bilirubin can rise when the albumin-binding sites are used up, increasing the risk of jaundice and ABE.

Bilirubin Toxicity

According to a summary of evidence collected by the Agency for Healthcare Research and Quality (AHRQ) (2002), term newborns without hemolysis are not at risk for brain damage or hearing impairment until serum bilirubin levels exceed 20 mg/dL. Factors influencing bilirubin toxicity to the brain cells of newborns are complex and incompletely understood; they include factors that affect the serum albumin concentration and factors that affect the binding of bilirubin to albumin, the penetration of bilirubin into the brain and the vulnerability of brain cells to the toxic effects of bilirubin. It is unknown at what level of bilirubin or under what circumstances significant risk of brain damage or ABE occurs, or when the risk of damage exceeds the risk of treatment. Concentrations considered toxic may vary in different ethnic groups and geographic locations. Neonates at risk for developing ABE have a history of acidosis, asphyxia, cold stress, prematurity and treatment with sulfonamides.

AHRQ (2002) identifies one issue that compounds the mystery of bilirubin toxicity: there is no consistent definition of clinically significant hyperbilirubinemia. Another issue is that most studies merge ethnic groups, gestational ages and feeding practices (breast or bottle).

Jaundice in Breastfeeding Infants

Jaundice associated with breastfeeding is characterized by an elevation in unconjugated bilirubin in otherwise healthy neonates. Two patterns of jaundice occur in breastfeeding infants: early-onset breastfeeding jaundice and late-onset breastmilk jaundice.

Early-onset breastfeeding jaundice, also called breastfeeding or breastfeeding-related jaundice, is more common and usually appears between 2 and 4 days of life. It may be related to increased enterohepatic shunting from decreased fluid intake and frequent feeding before maternal milk supply is established (Blackburn, 2007). Breastfed newborns with early-onset jaundice have bilirubin levels that are higher at 3 to 4 days and more likely to develop bilirubin levels in excess of 12 mg/dL than are bottle-fed newborns. Breastfed infants excrete less bilirubin in their stools than do formula-fed infants. The longer direct bilirubin remains in the intestine, the greater the probability that B-glucuronidase converts it back to indirect bilirubin. Decreased early stooling and a longer period to establish gut flora (needed for further breakdown and excretion of bilirubin in the intestine) are factors that can contribute to higher bilirubin levels in breastfed infants (Blackburn, 2007).

In late-onset breastmilk jaundice, the bilirubin level rises between the fourth and seventh day after birth, when physiologic jaundice is disappearing. It occurs in 1 in 100 to 200 breastfed infants and is related to components of breastmilk that interfere with bilirubin conjugation or excretion (Blackburn, 2007). Clinically, the infant with late-onset breastmilk jaundice appears yellow on day 5 to 6 of life; the jaundice gradually resolves by 3 months of age.

Support is mounting for increasing the frequency of breastfeeding as a measure to help reduce total bilirubin serum level (Bhutani, Johnson, Schwoebel & Gennaro, 2006; Hansen, 2006). Frequent breastfeeding (approximately ten feedings per 24-hour period) is associated with adequate milk volume and reduced serum bilirubin level. Early initiation and more frequent feedings also may increase stooling and increase fecal bilirubin clearance.

Screening and Diagnosis

Newborn jaundice can be detected by blanching the skin (AAP Subcommittee on Hyperbilirubinemia, 2004). As the total serum bilirubin level rises, jaundice develops in a cephalocaudal progression. There is yellowish discoloration of the sclerae, nails and skin. The nurse assesses the sclerae and skin over the forehead and trunk for jaundice every 4 to 8 hours and ensures that appropriate serum bilirubin monitoring is done, ideally upon visible recognition of signs of jaundice (Bhutani et al., 2006). Additional assessment should evaluate for bruising, activity level, feeding difficulties, behavior change and other signs of problems, including sepsis, hypoxia, asphyxia, hypoglycemia and hypothermia (Blackburn, 2007). Checking the maternal history for risk factors for jaundice allows for early risk identification and preparation.

AAP (2004) recommends that all infants be evaluated for jaundice by 24 hours if discharged before 24 hours of age, at 96 hours if discharged at 24 to 49.9 hours of age, or at 120 hours if discharged at 48 to 72 hours of age, with earlier and more frequent follow-up for infants at risk for hyperbilirubinemia. Risk should be considered based on any problems with cardiorespiratory instability, sepsis, thermal instability, poor nutrition or hydration, and lactation support (Bhutani et al., 2006). Table 48 identifies AAP's (2004) recommendations for evaluation and treatment of the healthy term newborn with hyperbilirubinemia.

Table 48. AAP Recommendations for Evaluation and Treatment of the Healthy Term Newborn with Hyperbilirubinemia
• Maternal/Perinatal testing should include ABO and Rh(D) typing and serum screen for unusual isoimmune antibodies.   • A direct Coombs test, blood typing and an Rh(D) type on cord blood should be done for mothers without prenatal care.   • Assessment of the infant should be performed when family history suggests the possibility of glucose-6-phosphate dehydrogenase deficiency or some other hemolytic disease.   • A total serum bilirubin should be drawn for infants jaundiced in the first 24 hours of life.   • If jaundice persists longer than 3 weeks, a measurement of total and direct serum bilirubin should be obtained.
AAP Subcommittee on Hyperbilirubinemia, 2004. Reproduced with permission from Pediatrics, 114, 297-316. © 2004 by the AAP.

Management

Therapeutic management of the infant with hyperbilirubinemia is based on clinical judgment, history, course and clinical findings. Providers always should consider potential benefits and risks of therapy.

Early postpartum discharge complicates management of jaundiced newborns because it places additional responsibilities on parents and guardians to recognize and respond to worsening jaundice or clinical signs. An indirect serum bilirubin level of 20 mg/dL is considered the upper limit, indicating immediate intervention if illness or associated conditions are present. The lower limit is 13 mg/dL. The infant should be assessed for a change in the CNS function, either depression or excitability.

Figure 6 provides the AAP Subcommittee on Hyperbilirubinemia (2004) algorithm for management of jaundice. Emphasis should be on prevention, rather than just treatment.

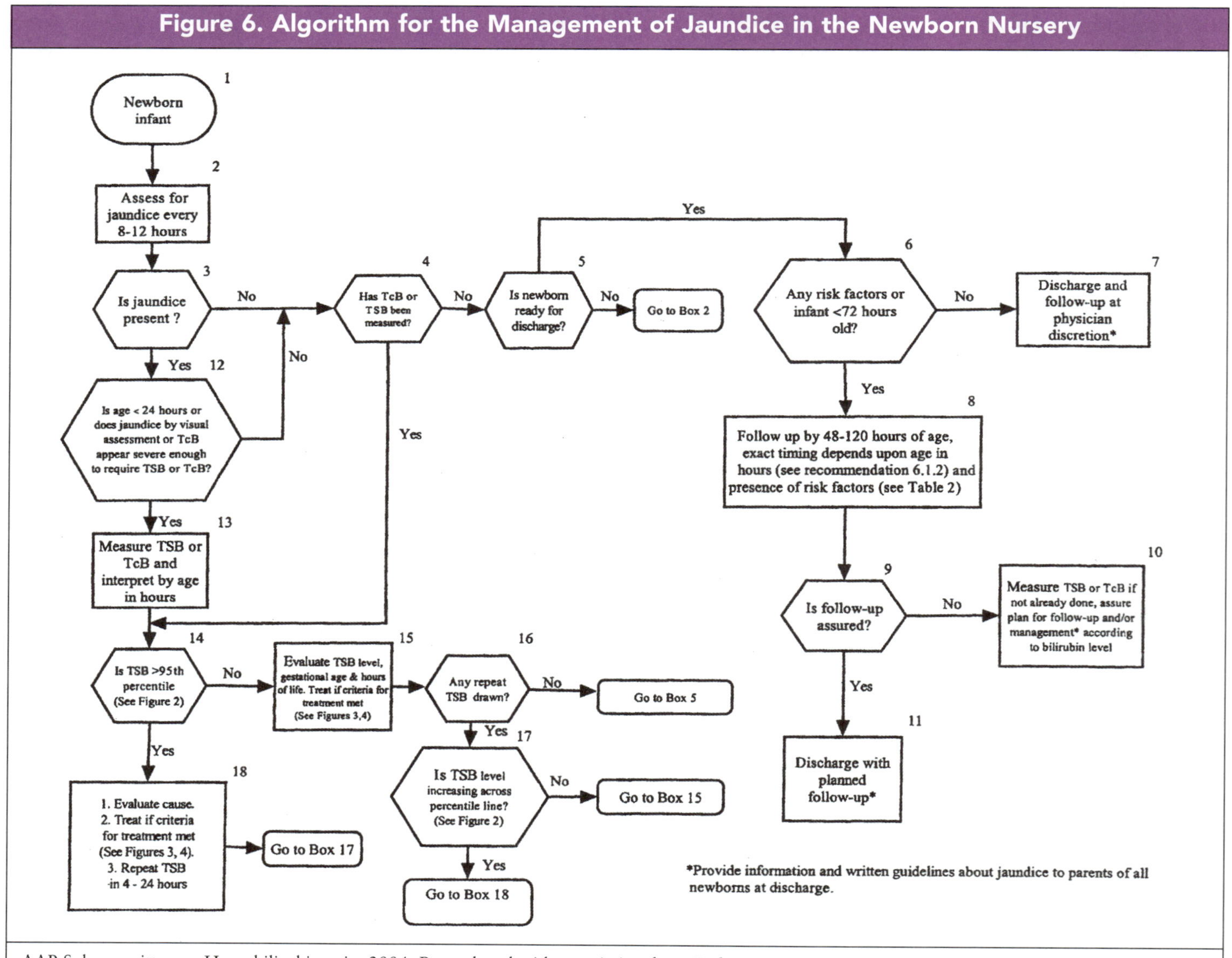

Figure 6. Algorithm for the Management of Jaundice in the Newborn Nursery

AAP Subcommittee on Hyperbilirubinemia, 2004. Reproduced with permission from *Pediatrics, 114,* 299. © 2004 by the AAP.

Phototherapy
Phototherapy is the application of fluorescent light on an infant's exposed skin. It is the most common treatment for hyperbilirubinemia. Phototherapy reduces bilirubin through photoisomerization and photo-oxidation, both of which convert bilirubin to a soluble form for excretion. Providers can deliver phototherapy with quartz lights, a bank of phototherapy lights or with fiberoptic blankets. All have advantages and disadvantages. The closer the light is to the skin's surface, the more intense the therapy; however, less skin surface is exposed and the greater the risk for burns. Table 49 identifies recommendations for phototherapy treatment. Table 50 identifies side effects of phototherapy.

Nursing care of infants receiving phototherapy involves assessment of physical and neurobehavioral status and interventions related to alterations in fluid volume, nutrition, skin integrity and thermal status. Injury prevention also is important. AAP Subcommittee on Hyperbilirubinemia (2004) recommends that a preventative approach be taken before discharge.

Parent Involvement and Education
Assessment of parental understanding of the neonate's condition and therapeutic needs is imperative. Nurses should give parents the opportunity to participate in parenting tasks, such as feeding, bathing and providing comfort to the newborn. The nurse should encourage questions and reinforce and clarify all information with parents. The nurse should discuss home management of mild to moderate physiologic jaundice, including frequency and volume of feedings, exposure to sunlight and follow-up serum testing programs. Parental teaching should address treatments resulting in bruising and genetic conditions that alter metabolism and might put their infant at greater risk for jaundice after discharge (Bhutani et al., 2006). Parents must know when to call for help or bring the infant in for follow-up care.

Postdischarge

Car Seats

One important measure parents can take to ensure the safety of their newborn is to position the infant in an approved safety seat each and every time they ride in a car. All states mandate the use of car seats for babies (March of Dimes, 2008). Although requirements may vary by state, a newborn must leave the hospital in a car seat. In many states, fire department personnel install seats for parents and instruct them on correct use.

The role of the car seat is to protect the infant from injury and/or death in motor-vehicle accidents. To prevent bradycardia, apnea and oxygen desaturation, parents should limit travel with their infant until he is able to hold his head up. If travel is necessary, one parent should ride in the back seat with the infant to watch for problems.

Bradycardia, apnea and oxygen desaturation also can occur when a baby is in an infant carrier or baby swing. Nurses should advise parents to avoid using these devices until the baby can hold his head up.

> **All states mandate the use of car seats for babies.**

Table 49. Recommendations for Phototherapy Treatment
• Ensure the infant is naked. Use diapers only if absolutely necessary and cut them to a minimum workable size.
• Protect the newborn's eyes with eye shields to reduce the risk of retinal damage. Ensure that the shield does not slip over the nose and obstruct the airway. Inspect the infant's eyes for injury every 4 to 8 hours with phototherapy lights off. Clean any discharge from the infant's eye with sterile water.
• Check the distance between the infant's skin and the light source using the manufacturer's guidelines. With fluorescent lamps, the distance should not be >50 cm (20 in). This distance may be reduced to 10 cm to 20 cm if temperature homeostasis is monitored to reduce the risk of overheating.
• Cover the inside of the bassinet with reflecting material. White linen works well. Hang a white curtain around the phototherapy unit and bassinet. These simple expedients can multiply energy delivery by several fold.
• When using spotlights, place the infant at the center of the circle of light because phototherapy drops off toward the circle's perimeter. Ensure that the infant does not move away from the high-energy area.
• Document the number of hours each lamp is used and change the lamps according to manufacturer's recommendations.
• Individualize timing of follow-up serum bilirubin testing. Monitor infants with extreme serum bilirubin values (>500 mmol/L or 30 mg/dL) every 1 to 2 hours. Monitor infants with moderate levels of serum bilirubin every 6 to 12 hours.
• Monitor the infant's hydration status by fluid and nutritional intake, urine and fecal loss, skin turgor, daily weights, serum electrolytes and urine-specific gravity. Adjust fluid intake accordingly. For infants who are fed orally, use breastmilk/formula because it serves as a vehicle to transport bilirubin out of the gut. Feed the newborn under phototherapy every 4 hours.
• Monitor the infant's thermal stability and temperature every 2 hours.
• Tailor expectations for efficacy of phototherapy to the infant's circumstances. For infants with rising serum bilirubin concentrations, a significant reduction in the rate of increase may be satisfactory. For infants in whom serum bilirubin concentrations are close to their peak, phototherapy should result in measurable reductions in serum bilirubin levels within a few hours. In general, the higher the starting serum bilirubin concentration, the more dramatic the initial rate of decline.
• Take individual circumstances into account when preparing to discontinue phototherapy. Discontinue phototherapy when serum bilirubin levels fall 25 mmol/L to 50 mmol/L or (1.5 mg/dL to 3 mg/dL) below the level that triggered the initiation of phototherapy. Serum bilirubin levels often rebound after treatment has stopped. Obtain follow-up tests within 6 to 12 hours after discontinuation.
• Use phototherapy only for infants who are clinically jaundiced. Prophylactic treatment is not indicated for infants who are not clinically jaundiced.
Altimier, Brown & Tedeschi, 2006; Hansen, 2006

Table 50. Side Effects of Phototherapy
• Thermal and other metabolic changes • Changes in fluid status with increased insensible water loss • Alteration in gastrointestinal function, activity and weight gain • Potential ocular effects related to lights and the use of eye coverings • Skin, hormonal and hematological changes • Psychobehavioral effects

Blackburn, 2007; Hansen, 2006

Back to Sleep: Sudden Infant Death Syndrome Prevention

Sudden infant death syndrome (SIDS) is the sudden death of an infant under 1 year of age which remains unexplained through case investigation, including performance of a complete autopsy, examination of the death scene and review of the clinical history (Willinger, James & Catz, 1991). In 2003, the SIDS rate for all races was 52.9 per 100,000 live births (Mathews, MacDorman & Menacker, 2002).

In 2005, the AAP Task Force on Infant Sleep Position and Sudden Infant Death Syndrome reviewed the evidence associated with SIDS-related issues and proposed new recommendations to reduce SIDS risk (Table 51). The Task Force also recommends continuing the *Back to Sleep* campaign with intensified public education for secondary caregivers (child care providers, grandparents, foster parents, babysitters) and focus on Black and American Indian/Alaska Native populations. Health care professionals in intensive-care and well-infant nurseries should implement *Back to Sleep* strategies well before anticipated discharge.

> Health care professionals in intensive-care and well-infant nurseries should implement *Back to Sleep* strategies well before anticipated discharge.

Table 51. AAP Recommendations to Reduce SIDS Risk
• Use *Back to Sleep*. Place infants on their back in supine positions (wholly on the back) for every sleep. • Use a firm sleep surface. Do not place soft materials or objects, such as pillows, quilts, comforters or sheepskins, under sleeping infants. • Keep loose bedding and soft objects, such as pillows, quilts, comforters, sheepskins and stuffed toys, out of an infant's sleeping environment. • Do not smoke during pregnancy. Maternal smoking during pregnancy has emerged as a major risk factor in almost every epidemiologic study of SIDS. • Maintain a separate, but proximate sleeping environment. The risk of SIDS is reduced when the infant sleeps in the same room as the mother. Use a crib, bassinet or cradle that conforms to the safety standards of the Consumer Product Safety Commission and the American Society for Testing and Materials. • Consider offering a pacifier at nap time and bedtime. The risk of SIDS is reduced with pacifier use during sleep. • Avoid overheating. Put the infant in light clothes for sleep. Keep the room temperature comfortable for a lightly clothed adult. • Avoid commercial devices marketed to reduce the risk of SIDS. There is no evidence that infants at a higher risk for SIDS can be identified by respiratory or cardiac monitoring. • Avoid development of positional plagiocephaly by utilizing "tummy time."

AAP Task Force on Infant Sleep Position and SIDS, 2005

Although multiple risk factors have been known for years (i.e., maternal smoking, prone sleeping), the importance of factors, such as soft bedding and covered airways, have been discovered more recently and are modifiable. Targeting education for staff and families can increase awareness and knowledge and change behaviors (Johanneman, Conkright, Warner, Altimier & Swehla, 2007).

Research shows that the advice of the infant's physician is most influential in determining the infant's sleep practices (AAP Task Force on Infant Sleep Position and SIDS, 2005). When a health care professional recommends the supine position to a parent, parents are more likely to place the infant supine than if they hadn't received the recommendation (Willinger, Ko, Hoffman, Kessler & Corwin, 2000). It is clear that all health care providers should discuss safe sleep practices with parents.

Back to Sleep has decreased the incidence of SIDS (AAP Task Force on Infant Sleep Position and SIDS, 2005). However, since the program began, the increase in supine positioning and the decrease in prone positioning have had consequences. For example, torticollis and plagiocephaly have increased and achievement of motor milestones has been delayed in healthy term infants (Chizawsky & Scott-Findlay, 2005). Infants may learn to crawl later because they are placed on their back in a supine position for most of the day and during sleep.

Skin Care and Bathing

Skin-care practices affect the neonate's overall health. Neonates require skin-care practices that optimize the skin's function as a barrier organ. Medical and nursing interventions related to skin are essential components of care.

Newborn skin is delicate and easily damaged (Tedeschi, 2007). Permeability increases as gestational age decreases. Caregivers should minimize the use of topical agents and cleanse the infant's skin gently with sterile water after applying antiseptic solutions to reduce absorption (AWHONN) & National Association of Neonatal Nurses [NANN], 2001). Alcohol is readily absorbed and may cause chemical damage. Bonding agents, such as benzoin, should be avoided because they increase the damage to skin when adhesives are removed. To remove adhesives, caregivers should use cotton soaked in sterile water, mineral oil or petrolatum, working gently from the edges of the adhesive; solvents, such as adhesive removers, should be avoided because they are readily absorbed through the skin. Caregivers should not remove adhesives until at least 24 hours after application, if possible, to allow the peak adhesive properties to diminish (Lund & Kuller, 2003). Stretchy cotton wraps may be used instead of tape to secure probes and electrodes (Altimier, Brown & Tedeschi, 2006; AWHONN & NANN, 2001).

Postmature infants are prone to skin breakdown. They have lost the protection of vernix in utero, and large areas of the stratum corneum may have shed because of damage from amniotic fluid. Generalized desquamation, areas of maceration, and cracks and fissures may be evident at birth. Scrubbing, peeling and lubrication should be avoided. Allowing natural regeneration of the skin is recommended (Blackburn, 2007).

An acid skin surface with a pH <5.0 is bactericidal and protects the skin from microbial invasion. Typically, skin pH becomes acidic after birth, forming an acid

When a health care professional recommends the supine position to a parent, parents are more likely to place the infant supine than if they hadn't received the recommendation.

mantle that defends against microorganisms. In a term neonate, the pH drops from a mean of 6.24 at birth to a mean of 4.94 in the first 4 days of life (Lund & Kuller, 2003). Higher skin pH allows bacteria to increase on the skin's surface, increasing the risk of infection. Bathing practices affect the skin's pH. The use of alkaline soaps disrupts the acid mantle and reduces its bactericidal quality.

Diaper rash, or diaper dermatitis, is common in neonates. It appears as red, excoriated areas of skin over the groin, thighs, perineum and buttocks caused by irritation from contact with urine and feces. Wetness, skin pH and the presence of enzymes in the stools contribute to diaper rash. Because skin already compromised by diaper rash is more susceptible to further injury and infection, diaper rash requires treatment. Frequent diaper changes, along with the application of zinc oxide, are recommended (AWHONN & NANN, 2001).

Abuse

Infant or child abuse is on the rise in the United States (National Center for Injury Prevention and Control [NCIPC], 2005). An estimated 1.98 children per 100,000 die from abuse or neglect each year; of these, 41 percent are <1 year of age (Walls, 2006). Table 52 lists common signs of neglect and abuse.

Table 52. Signs of Neglect and Abuse	
Common signs	<ul><li>Malnutrition</li><li>Bruising</li><li>Repeated fractures or fractures in various stages of healing</li><li>Intracranial hemorrhages</li><li>Retinal hemorrhages</li><li>Whiplash-like injuries, also called shaken baby syndrome (SBS)</li></ul>
Long-term signs	<ul><li>Irritability</li><li>Poor feeding</li><li>Listlessness</li><li>Inability to respond to stimuli, including talking, facial cues or touching</li><li>Seizures</li><li>Poor muscle tone</li><li>Failure to thrive</li><li>Apnea or bradycardia</li><li>Full fontanels</li><li>Posturing</li><li>Cognitive or developmental delays</li><li>Visual or hearing impairment (more likely with long-term than short-term abuse)</li></ul>

Walls, 2006

An estimated 1.98 children per 100,000 die from abuse or neglect each year; of these, 41 percent are <1 year of age.

SBS is caused by shaking or violent jerking of the upper body (Carbaugh, 2004). It occurs in about 1,000 to 1,500 infants and young children annually in the United States (NCIPC, 2005). It is estimated that 10 percent to 12 percent of all infant deaths from child abuse are caused by SBS (Altimier, 2008).

Risk Factors

Table 53 identifies risk factors for becoming an abuser. Men are more likely than women to abuse women and children (NCIPC, 2005); however, women are capable of abuse.

Table 53. Risk Factors for Becoming an Abuser
• Low frustration tolerance • Low socioeconomic status • Low education level • Living in unsafe neighborhood • Lack of social support • History of abuse during pregnancy (intimate partner violence) • History of mental illness • Teenage or immature parents • Parental substance abuse • Poor role models for parenting (Abusers may have been victims of physical, psychological or sexual abuse.) • Inexperience with child care • Unrealistic expectations of the child
Walls, 2006

Prevention

Nurses and other caregivers should watch for signs of potential abuse and direct parents to a variety of resources that help prevent abuse. Nurses should assess an infant's risk for abuse as well as teach parents before birth, after birth and after discharge about infant behavior and how to handle situations that lead to frustration. Table 54 summarizes the nurse's role in abuse prevention. The March of Dimes nursing module *Abuse During Pregnancy: A Protocol for Prevention and Intervention,* 3rd Edition (McFarlane, Parker & Moran, 2007) provides an overview of abuse prevention during pregnancy; many of the concepts presented in the module are applicable to abuse prevention after birth.

Table 54. The Nurse's Role in Abuse Prevention
• Identifying at-risk parents 　– History of abuse in the family 　– Alcohol or drug use 　– Overmedication with over-the-counter drugs 　– Abuse during pregnancy 　– An unwanted pregnancy/infant • Educating parents about abuse • Referring parents for counseling and services • Following up with parents or other family members
Walls, 2006

A number of organizations provide abuse-prevention resources for parents and caregivers. The National Center on Shaken Baby Syndrome (2006) (www.dontshake.com) offers information about abuse prevention and where parents can get help if they think their child has been abused. The center also offers programs geared specifically for dads and for middle and high school students. It's newest program for parents is the *Period of PURPLE* (**p**eak of crying, **u**nexpected crying, **r**esists soothing, **p**ain-like face, **l**ong-lasting crying, **e**vening crying) *Crying*. This program helps parents and caregivers understand the features of infant crying, especially inconsolable crying, that are frustrating and can lead to shaking or abuse. Additional parent resources are available from Bright Futures (www. brightfutures.org), Prevent Child Abuse America (www.preventchildabuse.org) and AAP (www.aap.org).

In 1989, the largest and best known SBS education and prevention program, *Don't Shake the Baby*, was targeted at new mothers in six Franklin County, Ohio hospitals (Showers, 1992a). Providers gave an information packet to new mothers and encouraged them to read the material. Packet distribution was timed with taking birth certificate information because it is when parents are focused on the infant's well-being and when they may understand and retain information most effectively. Mothers were asked to complete a response postcard aimed at assessing the effectiveness of the education program. According to monthly statistics provided by participating hospitals, a total of 15,708 births occurred during the period of the project. The project received response postcards from 3,293 parents, representing a 21 percent return rate. In response to a multiple-choice question, 98 percent of respondents selected the correct answer, "Shaking can cause brain damage or kill a baby." A new campaign called *Never Shake a Baby* uses brochures and cards describing strategies to manage crying infants and the parent's increasing level of frustration, informational videotapes about SBS, television and radio public service announcements, and posters for offices, classrooms and billboards (Showers, 1992b).

Summary

The term newborn is most often born healthy, making a complex but successful transition from fetus to newborn. Identifying risk in the newborn is enhanced by the availability of perinatal data, astute assessments during the immediate newborn period, and knowledge regarding expected norms and specific threats for newborns during the first days of life. Nursing assessments and interventions regarding transition to extrauterine life, glycemic control and thermoregulation are vital to newborn well-being and can significantly affect outcomes. Assessment of newborn behavior and function provide important information about the infant's transition period and ability to interact with the environment and caregivers. How an infant feeds, sleeps, wakes and responds indicate stability and well-being. Changes in these parameters may be early signs of problems.

Nurses who understand and can articulate the rationale for metabolic screenings, vitamin K prophylaxis and infection prevention can educate and provide anticipatory guidance to families. Knowledge about newborn jaundice helps facilitate timely and appropriate treatment and minimize complications. Discharge teaching includes infant readiness and safety, including car-seat safety, abuse prevention and other follow-up care.

Nurses contribute greatly to risk assessment and management during the immediate newborn period, minimizing the potential for complications and optimizing outcomes.

Clinical Application

The following activities will aid the learner in applying concepts presented in this module.

1. Assign an appropriate Apgar score to a newborn infant.

2. Determine appropriate gestational age and classify as SGA, AGA or LGA, based on physical and neurological assessment.

3. Review your institution's standard of care on thermal management of an infant receiving phototherapy in an incubator or warmer bed? Do these guidelines address thermoregulation? How?

4. Review your institution's standard of care for managing the neonate with hypoglycemia.

5. Identify resources in your community for follow-up management of hyperbilirubinemia in infants who are discharged early from the hospital.

6. Identify resources available for discharge teaching related to *Back to Sleep* and shaken baby syndrome?

Group Discussion Items

The following discussion items will aid the learner in applying concepts presented in this module.

1. Why is evidence-based practice important in today's health care environment?

2. Why is developmental care important to an infant and family's health?

3. What are infant states and how does your unit incorporate them into infant assessment?

4. Why is a family history important to a newborn's health?

5. What mechanisms are in place in your facility to prevent heat loss during delivery, in the first hour of life and during newborn assessment?

6. How are infants with hypoglycemia handled in your institution? What are the guidelines for management of infants with hypoglycemia and hyperglycemia?

7. How are infants with polycythemia managed in your facility?

8. What guidelines are available to monitor hyperbilirubinemia in the neonate discharged home?

9. What are four risk factors for infant abuse?

Slides

The following slides are provided for use with module group studies. Download slides from marchofdimes.com/nursingslides.

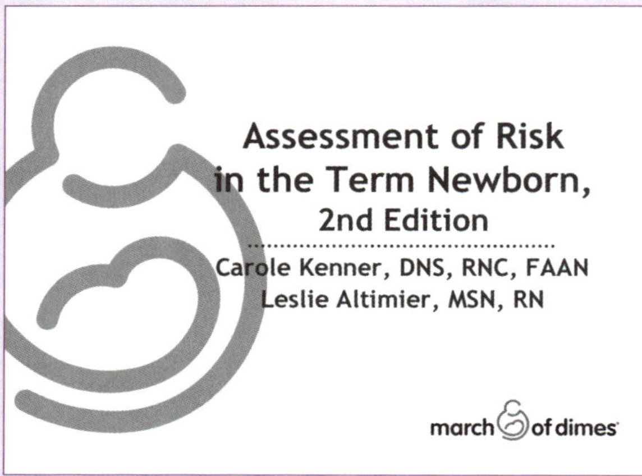

Slide 1

Transition from Fetal to Extrauterine Life

- Assessment and monitoring of neonatal adaptation are essential for early identification of problems.
- Nursing management during the early newborn period includes identification of risk factors, assessment, monitoring, intervention and postdischarge follow-up.

© 2008, March of Dimes

Slide 2

Evidence-based Practice (EBP) and Developmental Care

- EBP is based on the concept that care is grounded in research findings, rather than experience and tradition.
- Developmental care is individualized treatment based on diagnosis, gestational age and infant needs and capabilities.

© 2008, March of Dimes

Slide 3

Cardiovascular and Pulmonary Adaptation

- The most significant change at birth is that the lungs become the primary organ of oxygenation.
- When the umbilical cord is clamped, immediate circulatory changes occur because the placenta is no longer part of circulation.
- Nurses should evaluate and monitor any murmur or cyanosis in the neonate because they are signs of cardiovascular abnormalities (Lott, 2007).

© 2008, March of Dimes

Slide 4

Apgar Score

- Evaluates five physiologic signs at 1 minute and 5 minutes of life:
  - Heart rate
  - Respiration
  - Muscle tone
  - Reflex irritability
  - Color
- Assigns each sign a score of 0,1 or 2
- Is a convenient shorthand for reporting newborn status and response to resuscitation (AAP & ACOG, 2006)

© 2008, March of Dimes

Slide 5

Asphyxia

- Intrauterine asphyxia is the cessation of placental gas exchange that occurs before or during delivery. It is the most frequent cause of acidosis in the neonate and brain injury in the full-term newborn (Kenner & Lott, 2007).
- Perinatal asphyxia is failure of the newborn to establish adequate alveolar ventilation at birth . It is related to birth trauma, failed initiation of respiration, respiratory distress syndrome and apnea.

© 2008, March of Dimes

Slide 6

Delivery Management

- Ten percent of all newborns require some form of assistance at birth, and 1 percent require extensive resuscitation (Wu & Carlo, 2002).
- Discontinuation of resuscitation may be justified after 10 minutes of continuous and adequate resuscitation efforts if there are no signs of life (AAP & AHA, 2006).

© 2008, March of Dimes

Slide 7

Delivery Management (Continued)

- Suctioning may be done with a bulb syringe or a suction catheter.
- Meconium in the amniotic fluid complicates a small percentage of deliveries.
  - When a baby is born but not vigorous, endotracheal suctioning is required before the infant is dried or stimulated.

© 2008, March of Dimes

Slide 8

Effects of Anesthesia/Analgesia
(Mercer, Erickson-Owens, Graves & Haley, 2007)

- Most anesthesia and analgesia medications cross the placenta and enter fetal circulation in a dose-dependent fashion.
- Infants of mothers who receive narcotic analgesia or epidural anesthesia perform less well on tests of muscle tone, alertness and motor skills; however, these effects are transient.

© 2008, March of Dimes

Slide 9

Assessment of Gestational Age

- An accurate assessment incorporates size and maturity.
- Assessment methods include:
  - Mother's menstrual history
  - Prenatal ultrasonography
  - Evaluation of obstetric parameters
  - Postnatal maturational examinations
    - Dubowitz Assessment of Gestational Age
    - Lubchenco Scale
    - New Ballard Score

© 2008, March of Dimes

Slide 10

Infant Classification and Growth Assessment

- After assessing gestational age, the nurse plots the infant's length, weight and occipital-frontal head circumference (OFC) on intrauterine growth charts.
- Growth curves show measures of intrauterine growth in percentiles for each week of gestation.

© 2008, March of Dimes

Slide 11

Infant Classification and Growth Assessment (Continued)

Term	Percentile
Large for gestational age (LGA)	Above the 90th percentile
Appropriate for gestational age (AGA)	Between the tenth and 90th percentiles
Small for gestational age (SGA)	Below the tenth percentile

© 2008, March of Dimes

Slide 12

Physical Assessment

- Examination should occur within the first 24 hours of life after transition is complete (Verklan & Walden, 2004).
- Abnormal physical findings include:
  - Asymmetrical or weak movements
  - Floppy or rigid posture
  - High-pitched cry
  - Prolonged tremors
  - Inability to complete a full range of motion

© 2008, March of Dimes

Slide 13

Weight and Length (Kenner & Lott, 2007)

- An AGA term infant weighs 2,500 g to 4,000 g.
  - It is acceptable for infants to lose up to 10 percent of their birthweight in the first week of life.
  - Infants should return to their birthweight within the first 2 weeks of life.
- The term infant's length averages 45 cm to 55 cm.

© 2008, March of Dimes

Slide 14

Vital Signs (Kenner & Lott, 2007)

- The healthy infant has a respiratory rate between 40 and 60 breaths per minute.
- Heart rate should range from 120 to 160 beats per minute.
- Blood pressure ranges are related to gestational and chronologic ages.

© 2008, March of Dimes

Slide 15

Skin

Initial skin assessment includes:

- General color
- Consistency (smooth, peeling)
- Opacity
- Thickness
- Hair distribution
- Staining
- Epidermal consistency
- Obvious markings, moles or rashes

© 2008, March of Dimes

Slide 16

Head

- The average head circumference in a term infant is 35 cm; the customary range is 31 cm to 38 cm (Kenner & Lott, 2007).
- The infant has as many as six palpable fontanels at birth; the two most important are the anterior and posterior fontanels.

© 2008, March of Dimes

Slide 17

Face and Neck

- The nurse assesses:
  - The face for shape, symmetry, bruising and dysmorphic features
  - Gag, sucking and rooting reflexes
  - Facial movements for symmetry during crying
  - The neck for length, masses, webbing, mobility and the relationship of neck to body
- The nurse also performs detailed assessments of the ears, eyes, nose and mouth.

© 2008, March of Dimes

Slide 18

Thorax and Cardiovascular System

The nurse assesses:

- The infant's chest for size, symmetry, musculature, bony structure, number and location of nipples and ease of respiration
- The infant's heart for rate, rhythm, murmurs and character of sounds
- Femoral pulses in comparison with pulses in the upper extremities

© 2008, March of Dimes

Slide 19

Abdomen

- The nurse assesses the abdomen for contour, size, symmetry and umbilical cord location.
- The nurse palpates the abdomen to locate vital organs and any masses.
- The infant should urinate by 24 hours of age and have a bowel movement by 48 hours.

© 2008, March of Dimes

Slide 20

Kidneys

The nurse examines the kidneys for shape, texture and size (Altimier, Quatman & Howard, 2007):

- Kidneys are smooth and firm to touch when palpated.
- The length of the kidney in the term infant is 4.5 cm to 5.0 cm from the upper to the lower pole.

© 2008, March of Dimes

Slide 21

Anogenital Area and Genitalia

- The nurse evaluates the anus for patency and tone.
- In the male, the nurse checks the glans, urethral opening, prepuce and shaft of the penis; the scrotum is examined for size, rugation and the presence of testes.
- In the female, the nurse examines the labia, clitoris, urethral opening and external vaginal vault.

© 2008, March of Dimes

Slide 22

Skeletal System

- The nurse observes and palpates the curvature of the spine and performs passive flexion, extension and lateral bending.
- The nurse assesses extremities for symmetry, degree of flexion and presence of defects and fractures.

© 2008, March of Dimes

Slide 23

Sleep and Activity Patterns

The first 6 to 8 hours after birth are called the transitional period. During this period, the newborn experiences physiologic variations in three phases:

1. Reactivity immediately after birth
2. Relative inactivity
3. A second episode of reactivity

© 2008, March of Dimes

Slide 24

Infant State Assessment

- Evaluation of newborn behavior incorporates assessment of state, reactions to stimulation and the newborn's ability to move from one state to another.
- A state-organized infant can transition between states and has the physiological and behavioral ability to reach or withdraw from any state.

© 2008, March of Dimes

Slide 25

Newborn Screening and Genetic Testing

- The March of Dimes recommends newborn screening for 29 conditions (March of Dimes, 2006).
- Policies regarding parental informed consent for newborn screening differ by state.
- Sample collection for screening occurs between 48 and 72 hours after birth.

© 2008, March of Dimes

Slide 26

Thermoregulation

- Thermoregulation is the balance between heat production and heat loss.
- It is vital to the newborn and is entirely managed by nurses.
- It is closely linked to the infant's survival and health status (Kenner & Lott, 2007).

© 2008, March of Dimes

Slide 27

Heat Loss Mechanisms

- Conduction: transfer of heat when two solid objects are in surface-to-surface contact
- Convection: transfer of heat between areas that are in contact with each other but that are not solid
- Evaporation: heat loss caused by evaporation of water from the skin
- Radiation: transfer of heat from a warmer object to a cooler object without contact

© 2008, March of Dimes

Slide 28

Heat Dissipation

- Infants respond to overheating by vasodilation in the skin, which increases heat loss from the blood.
- In the first week of life, immaturity of the skin causes the largest amount of heat loss through evaporation.
- The newborn's head represents 21 percent of the total body surface area and accounts for a significant proportion of total heat loss (Blackburn, 2007).

© 2008, March of Dimes

Slide 29

Heat Production

The human body responds to cold in three ways:

1. Voluntary muscular activity (vasoconstriction and increased movement)
2. Shivering (inefficient in the term newborn)
3. Chemical or nonshivering thermogenesis (brown-fat metabolism for several hours after birth)

© 2008, March of Dimes

Slide 30

Temperature

- At birth, the neonate's temperature may decrease at a rate of 0.2 C to 1.0 C per minute, mainly through convective and evaporative heat loss.
- Norms (AAP & ACOG, 2007):
  - Rectal or auxiliary temperature of 36.5 C to 37.5 C
  - Skin temperature of 36 C to 36.5 C

Slide 31

Thermoneutral Environment

- A thermoneutral environment is a range of environmental temperatures in which an infant's metabolic rate is at a minimum and body temperature is maintained (Chandra & Baumgart, 2005b).
- At birth in a 25 C room, the infant requires 200 Kcal/kg/min to match the heat loss (Knobel, Wimmer & Holbert, 2005).

Slide 32

Temperature Assessment

- For neonates and infants, axillary temperatures closely correlate with rectal temperatures and are safer for the infant.
- Axillary temperature, on average, is 0.4 C less than rectal temperature (Kenner, 2003).

Slide 33

Hyperthermia

- Infant hyperthermia is caused by an overheated environment or fever.
  - In febrile infants, core temperature increases before skin temperature.
  - In an overheated environment, skin temperature increases first.
- Accurate documentation of skin, core and air temperatures can aid in the diagnosis.

Slide 34

Hypothermia

- One of the earliest signs of hypothermia is vasoconstriction.
- When a cold-stressed infant is rewarmed, skin temperature should not be warmer than core temperature by more than 1 C.
- The nurse slows the rewarming process if the infant becomes apneic or if blood pressure decreases.

Slide 35

Respiratory Distress

- Respiratory distress is a common neonatal complication that decreases oxygenation and carbon dioxide exchange.
- The three most common respiratory conditions that cause respiratory distress in the term newborn are:
  1. Pneumonia
  2. Transient tachypnea of the newborn (TTN)
  3. Meconium aspiration syndrome (MAS)

Slide 36

Hypoglycemia

- Caused by an inadequate supply of glucose, alterations in endocrine regulation or increased glucose regulation
- Can be transient or persistent and asymptomatic or symptomatic
- Usually defined as <35 mg/dL (Kenner & Lott, 2007); is not a single number—instead, is a trend of falling blood-glucose values

© 2008, March of Dimes

Slide 37

Hyperglycemia

- Usually is defined as a blood glucose level >125 mg/dL (whole blood) or 145 mg/dL to 150 mg/dL (plasma)
- Occurs most often in preterm newborns
- Is typically asymptomatic and detected on routine laboratory screening

© 2008, March of Dimes

Slide 38

Perinatal and Neonatal Infections

- The newborn's increased susceptibility to infection and decreased ability to respond to it make risk assessment and early intervention vital to reducing morbidity and mortality.
- Assessment of risk begins with a review of the maternal history and intrapartum record for evidence of maternal infection.

© 2008, March of Dimes

Slide 39

Predisposing Risk Factors for Newborn Infection

Maternal

• Malnutrition	• Vaginal colonization with GBS
• Lack of prenatal care	• Perineal colonization with E. Coli
• Substance abuse	• Prolonged rupture of membranes (>24 hours)
• TORCH infections	
• Peripartum maternal fever	• Sexually transmitted infection (STI)
• Clinical amnionitis	
• UTI at time of delivery	

Neonatal

• Prematurity	• IUGR
• Perinatal asphyxia	• Galactosemia
• Concurrent neonatal disease	• Congenital asplenia
	• Male sex

© 2008, March of Dimes

Slide 40

GBS

- GBS is a gram-positive, anaerobic bacterium that colonizes in the vagina or rectum of 10 percent to 30 percent of pregnant women (CDC, 2002).
- It is the most common cause of neonatal sepsis and meningitis in the United States (CDC, 2002).
- Treatment is with benzylpenicillin or ampicillin (Dear, 2005).

© 2008, March of Dimes

Slide 41

E. coli

- *E. coli* is a gram-negative rod that makes up most typical human fecal flora.
- It is the second most common cause of neonatal sepsis and meningitis in the United States (Dear, 2005).
- Treatment is with aminoglycoside alone or with cefotaxime if meningitis is suspected (Dear, 2005) .

© 2008, March of Dimes

Slide 42

Tuberculosis (TB)

- The incidence of TB in the United States has resurged since the late 1980s in association with the HIV epidemic (CDC, 2006c, 2006d).
- Transmission is by inhalation or ingestion of infected droplets, ingestion of infested breastmilk or contamination of traumatized skin or mucous membranes.

© 2008, March of Dimes

Slide 43

Tuberculosis (TB) (Continued)

- The Mantoux Purified Protein Derivative (PPD) skin test usually is positive once the infant develops antibodies to the bacilli.
- Infants are at minimal risk and require no anti-TB treatment if they are born to mothers who have completed treatment for TB and have no evidence of disease.

© 2008, March of Dimes

Slide 44

Sexually Transmitted Infections (STIs)

The CDC (2006b) suggests gathering information from clients about STIs using the five P's:

1. Partners
2. Prevention of pregnancy
3. Protection from STIs
4. Practices
5. Past history of STIs

© 2008, March of Dimes

Slide 45

Congenital Syphilis

- Syphilis can be transmitted across the placenta and through direct contact with active genital lesions during delivery.
- Evaluation for congenital syphilis includes physical examination and serologic testing.
- Nurses should examine cerebrospinal fluid in all infants born to mothers with syphilis during pregnancy and in those with suspected or proven congenital syphilis (Dear, 2005) .

© 2008, March of Dimes

Slide 46

Congenital Syphilis (Continued)

- Treatment at any stage is with parenteral penicillin G or benzylpenicillin (CDC, 2006c).
- Breastfeeding is not contraindicated for infants whose mothers have been treated.

© 2008, March of Dimes

Slide 47

Gonorrhea

- Intrapartum contamination usually occurs during contact with maternal secretions in the birth canal.
- It also can occur in utero after rupture of the membranes.

© 2008, March of Dimes

Slide 48

Gonorrhea (Continued)

- The most common clinical manifestation in neonates is ophthalmia neonatorum or conjunctivitis (CDC, 2006c).
- Correct administration of eye prophylaxis prevents gonococcal infection in most infants.
- There are no contraindications to breastfeeding with maternal gonococcal infection.

© 2008, March of Dimes

Slide 49

Hepatitis B (HBV)

- HBV is the hepatitis virus most often seen in perinatal and neonatal infection.
- Perinatal transmission is 76 percent in mothers with acute HBV in the third trimester and 10 percent in the first two trimesters (Dear, 2005).
- Ninety percent of infants born to women with HBV surface antigen and HBV envelop antigen are at risk for HBV during the first year of life (Kenner & Lott, 2007).

© 2008, March of Dimes

Slide 50

Hepatitis B (HBV) (Continued)

- Neonatal infection usually occurs at birth when the infant comes in direct contact with contaminated maternal blood and vaginal fluid.
- ACIP (2005) recommendations:
  - Infants born to HBV+ women
    - Dose 1 of HBIG vaccine at birth
    - Subsequent doses at 1 and 6 months (Pickering, 2006)
  - Infants born to non-HBV+ women
    - Dose 1 at birth or before discharge
    - Dose 2 at 1 or 2 months of age
    - Dose 3 at 6 to 18 months of age

© 2008, March of Dimes

Slide 51

HIV

- HIV is transmitted to the fetus in utero transplacentally, intrapartally through contact with maternal blood and in breastmilk.
- Infants usually develop signs and symptoms between 4 and 6 months of age with an incubation of 6 weeks to 10 years (CDC, 2006b, 2006c).

© 2008, March of Dimes

Slide 52

HIV (Continued)

- With proper screening and antiretroviral prophylaxis during labor and after birth, the risk for vertical transmission rate decreases (AAP & ACOG, 2007; Simpson, 2006).
- Research into pharmacological prevention in the neonate is promising, with clinical trials examining combinations of antiretroviral agents.

© 2008, March of Dimes

Slide 53

Chlamydia

- Chlamydia is the most widespread STI in the United States (Kenner & Lott, 2007).
- *Chlamydia trachomatis* is the bacterial agent most commonly found in perinatal infection (CDC, 2006c; Kenner & Lott, 2007).
- Transmission occurs at birth when the infant comes in contact with contaminated vaginal fluids in the birth canal.

© 2008, March of Dimes

Slide 54

Chlamydia (Continued)

- Acquisition occurs in approximately 50 percent of infants born vaginally to infected mothers and in some infants delivered by cesarean with intact membranes (Kenner & Lott, 2007).
- Breastfeeding is permitted unless antibiotics are used to treat maternal infection are contraindicated (Kenner & Lott, 2007).

© 2008, March of Dimes

Slide 55

Herpes Simplex (HSV)

- HSV-2 is the most common cause of disease in the newborn (Kenner & Lott, 2007).
- Transmission usually occurs intrapartally with ascending infection after rupture of membranes or through contact with an infected birth canal during vaginal delivery.

© 2008, March of Dimes

Slide 56

Herpes Simplex (HSV) (Continued)

- The risk of contracting the disease is 30 percent to 50 percent if the mother is experiencing a primary infection compared to <5 percent with a recurrent outbreak (Kenner & Lott, 2007).
- Treatment includes antiviral pharmacologic intervention with acyclovir and vidarabine.

© 2008, March of Dimes

Slide 57

TORCH Infections

- Toxoplasmosis
- Other infections (hepatitis B, syphilis, herpes zoster)
- Rubella (German measles)
- CMV
- Herpes

© 2008, March of Dimes

Slide 58

Vitamin K Deficiency

- One in 200 to 1 in 400 newborns not treated prophylactically with vitamin K at birth develop hemorrhagic disease of the newborn (HDN) (Blackburn, 2007).
- Every neonate should receive a single intramuscular dose of 0.5 mg to 1.0 mg of prophylactic vitamin K1 oxide at birth for prevention of early vitamin K deficiency bleeding (VKDB); parenteral vitamin K is required for late VKDB (AAP Committee on Fetus and Newborn, 2006).

© 2008, March of Dimes

Slide 59

Neonatal Polycythemia

- Neonatal polycythemia is a venous Hct of >65 percent or 22 g/dL (Blackburn, 2007).
- Increased blood viscosity is the underlying mechanism for clinically significant polycythemia.
- A screening Hct before 6 hours of age helps detect polycythemia and allows for appropriate management.

© 2008, March of Dimes

Slide 60

Jaundice

- More than half of all full-term newborns In the United States each year become clinically jaundiced (Hansen, 2006).
- There are three types of jaundice:
  1. Physiologic
  2. Pathologic
  3. Hyperbilirubinemia

© 2008, March of Dimes

Slide 61

Jaundice in Breastfeeding Infants

- Two patterns of jaundice can occur in breastfeeding infants:
  1. Late-onset breastmilk jaundice
  2. Early-onset breastfeeding jaundice
- Support is mounting for increasing the frequency of breastfeeding as a measure to help reduce total serum bilirubin level (Bhutani et al., 2006; Hansen, 2006).

© 2008, March of Dimes

Slide 62

Jaundice Screening and Diagnosis

- Newborn jaundice can be detected by blanching the skin (AAP, 2004).
- Nurses should assess the sclerae and skin over the forehead and trunk for jaundice every 4 to 8 hours and ensure that appropriate serum bilirubin monitoring is done (Bhutani et al., 2006).

© 2008, March of Dimes

Slide 63

Jaundice Management

- Phototherapy, the most common treatment for hyperbilirubinemia, reduces bilirubin through photoisomerization and photo-oxidation.
- Parents must know when to call for help or bring the infant in for follow-up care.

© 2008, March of Dimes

Slide 64

Car Seats

- All states mandate the use of car seats for babies (March of Dimes, 2008).
- A newborn must leave the hospital in a car seat.
- To prevent bradycardia, apnea and oxygen desaturation, parents should limit travel with their infant until he is able to hold his head up.

© 2008, March of Dimes

Slide 65

Sudden Infant Death Syndrome (SIDS)

- SIDS is the sudden death of an infant under 1 year of age which remains unexplained through case investigation, including performance of a complete autopsy, examination of the death scene and review of the clinical history.
- In 2003, the SIDS rate for all races was 52.9 per 100,000 live births (Mathews, MacDorman & Menacker, 2002).

© 2008, March of Dimes

Slide 66

SIDS Prevention (AAP Task Force on Infant Sleep Position and SIDS, 2005)

- Use *Back to Sleep*.
- Use a firm sleep surface.
- Keep loose bedding and soft objects out of the infant's sleeping environment.
- Do not smoke during pregnancy.
- Maintain a separate, but proximate sleeping environment.

© 2008, March of Dimes

Slide 67

SIDS Prevention (AAP Task Force on Infant Sleep Position and SIDS, 2005) (Continued)

- Consider offering a pacifier at nap time and bedtime.
- Avoid overheating
- Avoid commercial devices marketed to reduce the risk of SIDS.
- Avoid development of positional plagiocephaly by utilizing "tummy time."

© 2008, March of Dimes

Slide 68

Skin Care and Bathing

- Neonates require skin care practices that optimize the skin's function as a barrier organ.
- Skin pH becomes acidic after birth, forming an acid mantle that defends against microorganisms.
- Parents should use nonalkaline soaps when bathing their infant.

© 2008, March of Dimes

Slide 69

Signs of Abuse (Walls, 2006)

- Malnutrition
- Bruising
- Repeated fractures or fractures in various stages of healing
- Intracranial hemorrhages
- Retinal hemorrhages
- Whiplash-like injuries, also called shaken baby syndrome (SBS)

© 2008, March of Dimes

Slide 70

The Nurse's Role in Abuse Prevention (Walls, 2006)

- Identifying at-risk parents:
  - History of abuse in family
  - Alcohol or drug use
  - Overmedication with over-the-counter drugs
  - Abuse during pregnancy
  - An unwanted pregnancy/infant)
- Educating parents about abuse
- Referring parents for counseling and services
- Following up with parents or other family members

© 2008, March of Dimes

Slide 71

References

Advisory Committee on Immunization Practices (ACIP). (2005). A comprehensive immunization strategy to eliminate transmission of hepatitis B virus infection in the United States. *Mortality and Morbidity Weekly Report, 54*(rr16), 1-23.

Agency for Healthcare Research and Quality (AHRQ). (2002). Evidence report/technology assessment, number 65: *Management of neonatal hyperbilirubinemia*. [Online]. Available: www.ahrq. gov/clinic/epcsums/neonatalsum.htm

AIDS Education and Training Center (AETC) National Resource Center. (2006). *Guidelines for the use of antiretroviral agents in pediatric HIV infection*. Rockville, MD: Francois-Xavier Bagnoud Center, UMDNJ Health Resources and Services Administration, National Institutes of Health.

Altimier, L. (2004). Healing environment: For patients and providers. *Newborn and Infant Nursing Reviews. 4*(2), 89-92.

Altimier, L. (2008). Shaken baby syndrome. *Journal of Perinatal & Neonatal Nursing, 22*(1):68-76.

Altimier, L., Brown, B. & Tedeschi, L. (2006). *NANN guidelines for neonatal nursing policies, procedures, competencies and clinical pathways*. [Online]. Available: www.nann.org/i4a/store/category. cfm?category_id=77

Altimier, L., Quatman, A. & Howard, N. (2007). Genitourinary system. In L. Altimier (Ed.), *Mosby's neonatal nursing online course*. [Online]. Available: www.mcstrategies.com/media/nursing_neonatal.pdf

American Academy of Pediatrics (AAP) & American College of Obstetricians and Gynecologists (ACOG). (2007). *Guidelines for perinatal care* (6th ed.). Washington, DC: Author.

American Academy of Pediatrics (AAP) & American Heart Association (AHA). (2006). *Textbook of neonatal resuscitation* (5th ed.). Elk Grove Village, IL: Author.

American Academy of Pediatrics (AAP) Committee on Fetus and Newborn. (2006). AAP policy: Controversies concerning vitamin K and the newborn. *Pediatrics, 112,* 191-192.

American Academy of Pediatrics (AAP) Committee on Fetus and Newborn & American College of Obstetricians and Gynecologists (ACOG) Committee on Obstetric Practice. (1996). Use and abuse of the Apgar score. *Pediatrics, 98,* 141-142.

American Academy of Pediatrics (AAP) Committee on Fetus and Newborn & the American College of Obstetricians and Gynecologists (ACOG) Committee on Obstetrical Practice. (2006). Policy statement: The APGAR score. *Advances in Neonatal Care, 6*(4), 220-223.

American Academy of Pediatrics (AAP) Subcommittee on Hyperbilirubinemia. (2004). Clinical practice guideline: Management of hyperbilirubinemia in the newborn infant 35 weeks or more of gestation. *Pediatrics, 114,* 297-316.

American Academy of Pediatrics (AAP) Task Force on Infant Sleep Position and Sudden Infant Death Syndrome (SIDS). (2005). The changing concept of sudden infant death syndrome: Diagnostic coding shifts, controversies regarding the sleep environment, and new variables to consider in reducing risk. *Pediatrics, 116*(5), 1245-1255.

American Heart Association (AHA). (2005). Guidelines for cardiopulmonary resuscitation and emergency cardiovascular care. Part 13: Neonatal resuscitation guidelines. *Circulation, 112* (suppl IV), 188-195.

Apgar, V. (1953). A proposal for a new method of evaluation of the newborn infant. *Current Researches Anesthesia and Analgesia, 32,* 260-267.

Association of Women's Health, Obstetric & Neonatal Nurses (AWHONN). (2004). *National standards for newborn screenings*. Washington, DC: Author.

Association of Women's Health, Obstetric and Neonatal Nurses (AWHONN) & National Association of Neonatal Nurses (NANN). (2001). *Evidence-based clinical practice guideline: Neonatal skin care*. Washington, DC: Author.

Avery, M.E., Gatewood, O.B. & Brumley, G. (1966). Transient tachypnea of newborn. Possible delayed resorption of fluid at birth. *American Journal of Diseases of Children, 111*(4), 380-385.

Babson, S.G., Behrman, R.E. & Lessel, R. (1970). Liveborn birthweights for gestational age of white middle class infants. *Pediatrics, 45*, 937-944.

Ballard, J.L., Khoury, J.C., Wedig, K., Wang, L., Eilers-Walsman, B.L. & Lipp, R. (1991). New Ballard score, expanded to include extremely premature infants. *Journal of Pediatrics, 119*, 417–423.

Ballard, J.L., Novak, K.K. & Driver, M.A. (1979). A simplified score for assessment of fetal maturation of newly born infants. *Journal of Pediatrics, 95*(6), 769-774.

Barnett, E. & Klein, J.O. (2006). Bacterial infections of the respiratory tract. In J.S. Remington, J.O. Klein, C.B. Wilson & C.J. Baker (Eds.), *Infectious diseases of the fetus and newborn infant* (6th ed., pp. 297-317). Philadelphia: W.B. Sanders.

Barron, M.L. (2007). *Antepartum assessment and laboratory evaluation: The first visit.* [Online]. Available: www.marchofdimes.com/nursing

Battaglia, F.C. & Lubchenco, L.O. (1967). A practical classification of newborn infants by weight and gestational age. *Journal of Pediatrics, 71*, 159-163.

Bhutani, V.K., Johnson, L.H., Schwoebel, A. & Gennaro, S. (2006). A systems approach for neonatal hyperbilirubinemia in term and near-term newborns. Journal of Obstetric, *Gynecologic & Neonatal Nursing, 35*(4), 444-455.

Blackburn, S. T. (2003). *Maternal, fetal, and neonatal physiology: A clinical perspective* (2nd ed). Philadelphia: W.B. Saunders.

Blackburn, S.T. (2007). *Maternal, fetal, and neonatal physiology: A clinical perspective* (3rd ed.). Philadelphia: W.B. Saunders.

Blackburn, S. & Bakewell-Sachs, S. (2004). *Understanding the behavior of term infants.* [Online]. Available: www.marchofdimes.com/nursing

Blackburn, S. & Bakewell-Sachs, S. (2007). *Understanding your newborn: An interactive program for new parents.* [Online]. Available: www.marchofdimes.com/newborn

Brazelton, T.B. (1984). *Neonatal behavioral assessment scale* (2nd ed.). Philadelphia: J.B. Lippincott.

Brown, B. (2007). Newborn Assessment. In L. Altimier (Ed.), *Mosby's neonatal nursing online course.* [Online). Available: www.mcstrategies.com/media/nursing_neonatal.pdf

Brozanski, B.S., Jones, J.G., Krohn, M.J. & Jordan, J.A. (2006). Use of polymerase chain reaction as a diagnostic tool for neonatal sepsis can result in a decrease in use of antibiotics and total neonatal intensive care unit length of stay. *Journal of Perinatology, 26*(11), 688-692.

Carbaugh, S.F. (2004). The long road home. Understanding shaken baby syndrome. *Advances in Neonatal Care, 4*, 105-117.

Centers for Disease Control & Prevention (CDC). (2002). Prevention of perinatal group B streptococcal disease: Revised guidelines from CDC. *Morbidity and Mortality Weekly Reports, 51*(rr11), 1-22.

Centers for Disease Control & Prevention (CDC), National Office of Public Health Genomics (2006a). *Family history as a tool for public health and preventive medicine: A public health perspective.* [Online]. Available: www.cdc.gov/genomics/training/perspectives/famhistr.htm

Centers for Disease Control & Prevention (CDC). (2006b). *Sexually transmitted diseases treatment guidelines.* [Online]. Available: www.cdc.gov/mmwr/preview/mmwrhtml/rr5511a1.htm

Centers for Disease Control & Prevention (CDC). (2006c). Revised recommendations for HIV testing of adults, adolescents and pregnant women in health-care settings. *Mortality and Morbidity Weekly Report Recommendations and Reports, 55*(rr14), 1-17.

Centers for Disease Control & Prevention (CDC). (2006d). *U.S. tuberculosis cases at an all-time low in 2005 but drug resistance increasing.* [Online]. Available: www.cdc.gov/OD/OC/MEDIA/pressrel/fs060323.htm

Centers for Disease Control & Prevention (CDC). (2007). *Early hearing detection and intervention program.* [Online]. Available: www.cdc.gov/ncbddd/ehdi/default.htm

Chandra, S. & Baumgart, S. (2005a). Fetal and neonatal thermoregulation. In A.R. Spitzer (Ed.). *Intensive care of the fetus & neonate* (2nd ed., pp. 495–513). Philadelphia: Elsevier.

Chandra, S. & Baumgart, S. (2005b). Temperature regulation of the premature infant. In H. Taeusch, R.A. Ballard & C.A. Gleason (Eds.). *Avery's diseases of the newborn* (8th ed., pp. 364–371). Philadelphia: Elsevier.

Chizawsky, L.L. & Scott-Findlay, S. (2005). Tummy time! Preventing unwanted effects of the "Back to Sleep" campaign. *AWHONN Lifelines, 9*(5), 382-387.

Cooper, L.Z. & Alford, C.A. (2006). Rubella. In J.S. Remington, J.O. Klein, C.B. Wilson & C.J. Baker (Eds.), *Infectious diseases of the fetus and newborn infant* (6th ed., pp. 893-926) . Philadelphia: W.B. Saunders.

Cronenwett, L. (2002). Research, practice and policy: Issues in evidence-based care. *Online Journal of Issues in Nursing.* [Online]. Available: nursingworld.org/OJIN/KEYNOTES/speech_2.htm

Crowenwett, L., Sherwood, G., Barnsteiner, J., Disch, J., Johnson, J., Mitchell, P., et al. (2007). Quality and safety education for nurses. *Nursing Outlook, 5S*(3), 122-31.

Dear, P. (2005). Infection in the newborn. In J.M. Rennie (Ed.), *Robertson's textbook of neonatology* (4th ed., pp. 1011-1092). London: Elsevier/Churchill Livingstone.

Dodd, V. (1966). Gestational age assessment. *Neonatal Network, 15*(1), 27-36.

Dubowitz, L.M.S., Dubowitz, V. & Goldberg, C. (1970). Clinical assessment of gestational age in the newborn infant. *Journal of Pediatrics, 77*(1), 1-10.

du Plessis, A.J. (2005). Perinatal asphyxia and hypoxic-ischemic brain injury in the full-term infant. In A.R. Spitzer (Ed.), *Intensive care of the fetus & neonate* (2nd ed., pp. 775-793). Philadelphia: Elsevier.

Erdman, S. & Erdman, T. (2007). Gastrointestinal system. In L. Altimier (Ed.), *Mosby's neonatal nursing online course.* [Online]. Available: www.mcstrategies.com/media/nursing_neonatal.pdf

Fenton, T.R. (2003). Licensee Biomed Central Ltd. [Online]. Available: www.biomedcentral.com/1471-2431/3/13

Figueroa, R., Khabbaz, A.A. & Quirk, J.G. (2005). Identification and management of the fetus at risk for acidosis. In A.R. Spitzer (Ed.), *Intensive care of the fetus & neonate* (2nd ed., pp. 91-110). Philadelphia: Elsevier.

Flenady, V.J. & Woodgate, P.G. (2003). Radiant warmers versus incubators for regulating body temperature in newborn infants. *Cochrane Database of Systematic Reviews,* (2):CD000435.

Fuloria, M. & Wiswell, T.E. (2005). Meconium and the compromised fetus and neonate. In A.R. Spitzer (Ed.), *Intensive care of the fetus & neonate* (2nd ed., pp. 375-383). Philadelphia: Elsevier.

Gamblian, V.W., Weiland, J. & Park, N.C. (2003). Assessment and management of the endocrine system. In C. Kenner & J. Lott (Eds.), *Comprehensive neonatal nursing* (3rd ed., pp. 531-549). St. Louis: Saunders.

Gartner, M. & Hollander, M. (1972). Disorders of bilirubin metabolism. In N.S. Assali (Ed.), *Pathophysiology of Gestation* (Vol. 3, 457). **NEED CITY:** Academic Press.

Guthrie, R. & Susi, A. (1963). A simple phenylalanine method for detecting phenylketonuria in large populations of newborn infants. *Pediatrics, 32,* 338-343.

Hansen, T.W.R. (2006). *Neonatal jaundice.* [Online]. Available: www.emedicine.com/ped/topic1061.htm

Hegyi, T., Carbone, M.T., Anwar, M., Ostfeld, B., Hiatt, M., Koons, A.A., et al. (1994). Blood pressure ranges in premature infants, I: The first hours of life. *Journal of Pediatrics, 124,* 627-633.

Holditch-Davis, D., Blackburn, S.T. & VandenBerg, K. (2003). Newborn and infant neurobehavioral development. In C. Kenner & J. Lott (Eds.), *Comprehensive neonatal nursing* (3rd ed., pp. 236-284). St. Louis: Saunders.

Institute of Medicine (IOM). (2001). *Envisioning the national health care quality report.* Washington, DC: National Academies Press.

Institute of Medicine (IOM). (2003). *Health professions education: A bridge to quality.* Washington, DC: National Academies Press.

Jain, L. & Eaton, D.C. (2006). Physiology of fetal lung fluid clearance and the effect of labor. *Seminars in Perinatology, 30*(1), 34-43.

Johannemann, T., Conkright, L., Warner, B., Altimier, L. & Swehla, M. (2007). Safe sleep: One organization's approach to enhancing patient safety. *Newborn and Infant Nursing Reviews, 7*(2).

Katz, L.L. & Stanley, C. (2005). Disorders of glucose and other sugars. In A.R. Spitzer (Ed.), *Intensive care of the fetus & neonate* (2nd ed., pp. 1167-1178). Philadelphia: Elsevier.

Kendrick, J.M. (2004). *Diabetes in pregnancy* (3rd ed.). New York: March of Dimes.

Kenner, C. (2003). Neonatal thermoregulation. In C. Kenner & J.W. Lott (Eds.), *Comprehensive neonatal nursing: A physiologic perspective* (3rd ed., pp. 212-217). Philadelphia: W.B. Saunders.

Kenner, C. & Lott, J.W. (Eds.). (2007). *Comprehensive neonatal care: A physiologic perspective* (4th ed.). Philadelphia: W.B. Saunders.

Kenner, C. & Moran, M.B. (2005). Screening and genetic testing. *Journal of Midwifery & Women's Health, 50*(3), 219-226.

Knobel, R.B., Wimmer, J.E. & Holbert, D. (2005). Heat loss prevention for preterm infants in the delivery room. *Journal of Perinatology, 25*(5), 304-308.

Lessaris, K.J. (2005). Polycythemia of the newborn. [Online]. Available: www.emedicine.com/ped/topic2479.htm

Lopriore, E., van Burk, F., Walther, F. & Arnout, J. (2004). Correct use of the Apgar score for the assessment of the newborn babies: Questionnaire study. *British Medical Journal, 329,* 143-144.

Lott, J. (2007). Cardiac system. In L. Altimier (Ed.), *Mosby's neonatal nursing online course.* [Online]. Available: www.mcstrategies.com/media/nursing_neonatal.pdf

Louw, R. & Maree, C. (2005). The effect of formal exposure to developmental care principles on the implementation of developmental care positioning and handling of preterm infants by neonatal nurses. *Health, 10*(2), 24-32.

Lubchenco, L.O., Searls, D.T. & Brazie, J.V. (1972). Neonatal mortality rate: Relationship to birthweight and gestational age. *Journal of Pediatrics, 81,* 814-822.

Lund, C.H. & Kuller, J.M. (2003). Assessment and management of the integumentary system. In C. Kenner & J.W. Lott (Eds.), *Comprehensive neonatal nursing: A physiologic perspective* (pp. 700-724). Philadelphia: W.B. Saunders.

March of Dimes. (2008) *Car seats.* [Online]. Available: http://www.marchofdimes.com/pnhec/298_1041.asp

March of Dimes. (2006). *Recommended newborn screening tests: 29 disorders.* [Online]. Available: www.marchofdimes.com/professionals/14332_15455.asp

Matthews, T.J., MacDorman, M.F. & Menacker, F. (2002). Infant mortality statistics from the 1999 period linked birth/infant death data set. *National Vital Statistics Reports, 50*(4), 1-27.

McFarlane, J., Parker, B. & Moran, B.A. (2007). *Abuse during pregnancy: A protocol for prevention and intervention* (3rd ed.). White Plains, NY: March of Dimes Foundation.

McGowan, J., Hagedohn, M.L. & Hay, W.W., Jr. (1998). Glucose homeostasis. In G.B. Merenstein & S.L. Gardner (Eds.), *Handbook of neonatal intensive care* (4th ed., pp. 259-275), St. Louis: Mosby.

Melnyk, B.M. & Fineout-Overholt, E. (2005). *Evidence-based practice in nursing & healthcare: A guide to best practice.* Philadelphia: Lippincott, Williams & Wilkins.

Melnyk, B.M. (2007, March 10). *Dream Big: Putting EBP into practice.* Presented at the University of Oklahoma College of Nursing, Oklahoma City, OK.

Mercer, J.S., Erickson-Owens, D.A., Graves, B. & Haley, M.M. (2007). Evidence-based practices for the fetal to newborn transition. *Journal of Midwifery & Women's Health.* 52(3):262-272.

Merck & Co. (2005). Perinatal tuberculosis (TB). *Merck manuals online medical library.* [Online]. Available: www.merck.com/mmpe/sec19/ch279/ch279n.html

Merrill, J.D. & Ballard, R.A. (2005). Resuscitation in the delivery room. In H. Taeusch, R.A. Ballard & C.A. Gleason (Eds.), *Avery's diseases of the newborn* (8th ed., pp. 349-363). Philadelphia: Elsevier.

Morris, A.C. (2007a). Meconium aspiration syndrome. In L. Altimier (Ed.), *Mosby's neonatal nursing online course.* [Online]. Available: www.mcstrategies.com/media/nursing_neonatal.pdf

Morris, A.C. (2007b). Persistent pulmonary hypertension of the newborn. In L. Altimier (Ed.), *Mosby's neonatal nursing online course.* [Online]. Available: www.mcstrategies.com/media/nursing_neonatal.pdf

National Center on Shaken Baby Syndrome. (2006). *Parents, family and friends.* [Online]. Available: www.dontshake.com/Audience.aspx?CategoryID=1

National Center for Injury Prevention and Control (NCIPC). (2005). *Child maltreatment: Fact sheet.* [Online]. Available: www.cdc.gov

National Institute of Child Health and Human Development (NICHD) and National Institute of Allergy and Infectious Diseases (NIAID). (2006). *Trial of three neonatal antiretroviral regimens for prevention of intrapartum HIV transmission.* [Online]. Available: www.clinicaltrials.gov/ct/show/NCT00099359;jsessionid=BEF16396CC4C00C5B9C471D7EE079FAF?order=2

National Newborn Screening and Genetics Resource Center (NNSGRC). (1997). *Newborn screening.* [Online]. Available: genes-r-us.uthscsa.edu/resources/consumer/statemap.htm

Oh, W. (1982). Neonatal polycythemia and hyperviscosity. *Pediatric Clinics of North America, 33,* 523.

Pickering, L.K. (Ed.). (2006). *Red book: 2006 Report of the committee on infectious diseases* (27th ed.). Elk Grove Village, IL: American Academy of Pediatrics.

Puckett, R.M. & Offringa, M. (2006). Prophylactic vitamin K for vitamin K deficiency bleeding in neonates (Cochrane Review). *The Cochrane Library, 3.*

Risken, A., Abend-Weinger, M., Riskin-Mashiah, S., Kugelman, A. & Bader, D. (2005). Cesarean section, gestational age and transient tachypnea of the newborn: Timing is the key. *American Journal of Perinatology, 22*(7), 377-382.

Shankaran, S., Laptook, A.R., Ehrenkranz, R.A., Tyson, J.E., McDonald, B.S., Donovan, E.F., et al. (2005). Whole-body hypothermia for neonates with hypoxic-ischemic encephalopathy. *New England Journal of Medicine, 353,* 1574-1584.

Showers, J. (1992a). Don't shake the baby: Effectiveness of a prevention program. *Child abuse and Neglect,* 15:11-18.

Showers, J. (1992b). Shaken baby syndrome: The problem and a model for prevention. *Children Today,* 21:34-37.

Simpson, K.R. (2006). Prevention of perinatal transmission of HIV. *MCN: The American Journal of Maternal Child Nursing, 31*(6), 396.

Stanley, C.A. & Pallotto, E.K. (2005). Disorders of carbohydrate metabolism. In H. Taeusch, R.A. Ballard & C.A. Gleason (Eds.). *Avery's diseases of the newborn* (8th ed., pp. 1410-1418). Philadelphia: Elsevier.

Sundaravaradan, V., Saxena, S.K., Ramakrishnan, R., Yedavalli, V.R.K., Harris, D.T. & Ahmad, N. (2006). Differential HIV-1 replication in neonatal and adult blood mononuclear cells is influenced at the level of HIV-1 gene expression. *Proceeding of the National Academy of Sciences of the United States of America, 103*(31), 11701-11706.

Tappero, E. & Honeyfield, M.E. (2003). *Physical assessment of the newborn: A comprehensive approach to the art of physical examination.* Santa Rosa, CA: NICU Ink.

Tedeschi, L. (2007). Integumentary system. In L. Altimier (Ed.), *Mosby's neonatal nursing online course.* [Online]. Available: www.mcstrategies.com/media/nursing_neonatal.pdf

Theroux, R. (2006). How to bring evidence into your practice. *AWHONN Lifelines, 10*(3), 244-249.

Uebel, P. (2007). Thermoregulation. In L. Altimier (Ed.), *Mosby's neonatal nursing online course.* [Online]. Available: www.mcstrategies.com/media/nursing_neonatal.pdf

Verklan, T. & Walden, M. (2004). *Core curriculum for neonatal intensive care nursing* (3rd ed.). St. Louis: W.B. Saunders.

Waitzman, K. (2007). Neuromotor development. In L. Altimier (Ed.), *Mosby's neonatal nursing online course.* St. Louis, MO: Elsevier. [Online]. Available: www.mcstrategies.com/media/nursing_neonatal.pdf

Walls, C. (2006). Shaken baby syndrome education: A role for nurse practitioners working with families of small children. *Journal of Pediatric Health Care, 20*(5), 304-310.

Willinger, M., James, L.S. & Catz, C. (1991). Defining the Sudden Infant Death Syndrome SIDS: Deliberations of an expert panel convened by the National Institute of Child Health and Human Development. *Fetal and Pediatric Pathology, 11*(5): 677-84.

Willinger, M., Ko C-W, Hoffman, H.J., Kessler, R.C. & Corwin, M.J. (2000). Factors associated with caregivers' choice of infant sleep position, 1994-1998: The national infant sleep position study. *Journal of the American Academy of Medicine, 283,* 2135-2142.

Wu, T.J. & Carlo, W.A. (2002). Neonatal resuscitation guidelines 2000: Framework for practice. *Journal of Maternal, Fetal and Neonatal Medicine, 11*(1), 2-3.

Zaichkin, J. (2006). NRP 2006: What you should know. *Neonatal Network, 25*(2), 145-151.

Supplementary Materials

Books and Journals

Altimier, L. (Ed.) *Newborn and Infant Nursing Reviews.*
Philadelphia: W.B. Saunders (published quarterly).

Kenner, C., McGrath, J. & National Association of Neonatal Nurses (NANN).
(2004). *Developmental care of newborns and infants: A guide for health
professionals.* St. Louis: Mosby.

Web Sites

American Academy of Pediatrics (AAP)
www.aap.org
Neonatal Resuscitation Program
www.aap.org/nrp
AAP policy statements
aappolicy.aappublications.org

Bright Futures
www.brightfutures.org

Centers for Disease Control and Prevention (CDC)
www.cdc.gov
Morbidity and Mortality Weekly Reports
www.cdc.gov/mmwr
Newborn screening
www.cdc.gov/nceh/dls/newborn_screening.htm

Council of International Neonatal Nurses (COINN)
www.coinnurses.org

Healthy Families America
www.healthyfamiliesamerica.org

March of Dimes
marchofdimes.com

National Association of Neonatal Nurses (NANN)
www.nann.org

National Center on Shaken Baby Syndrome
www.dontshake.com

Neonatology on the Web
www.neonatology.org

Prevent Child Abuse America
www.preventchildabuse.org

Recommended Standards for Newborn ICU Design
www.nd.edu/~nicudes

Zero to Three
www.zerotothree.org